Slim And Savory Diet Cookbook 2024

Unleash Long-Term Vitality with Easy, Tasty, and Nutrient-Packed Recipes

Evelyn G. Powell

Copyright

Disclaimer

The content in this cookbook is intended for general informative purposes only. While every effort has been made to ensure the accuracy and completeness of the content, Evelyn G. Powell, the publisher, and contributors cannot be held responsible for any errors, omissions, or outcomes related to the use of the information contained in this book.

The recipes, tips, and nutritional information are not intended to be a substitute for professional dietary or medical advice. Readers are encouraged to consult with a qualified healthcare professional or nutritionist regarding individual dietary needs, restrictions, or health conditions.

Evelyn G. Powell, the author, and the publisher disclaim responsibility for any adverse effects resulting directly or indirectly from the information provided in this cookbook. Cooking techniques, ingredient availability, and nutritional values may vary, and readers should use their discretion and judgment when preparing and consuming recipes.

By using this cookbook, readers agree to release Evelyn G. Powell, the author, the publisher, and contributors from any liability related to the use or misuse of the information provided herein. Cooking is a creative and subjective activity, and individual preferences and dietary needs may vary.

About the author

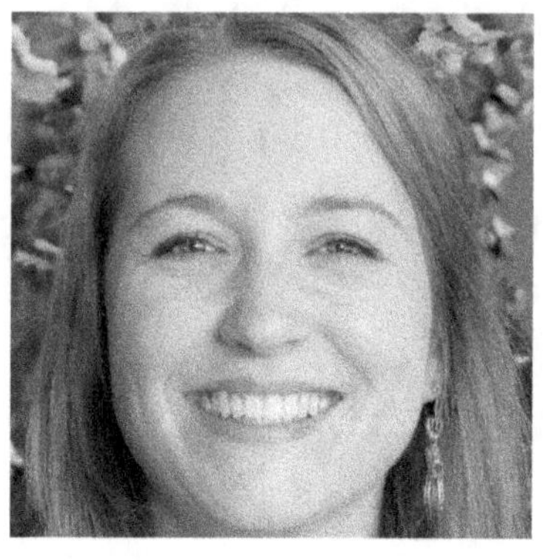

Meet the mastermind behind these scrumptious recipes - Evelyn G. Powell. She does more than cook; she's a culinary maestro, and her kitchen is where the magic occurs!

Every sizzle and stir in Evelyn's kitchen is an expression of her passion for cooking.
She has an inventive brain that will not be held back. Her recipes aren't just about flavors; they're accounts of culinary advancement and trying investigation.

However, it goes beyond taste; Evelyn is about balance. Her creations transform ordinary ingredients into extraordinary experiences by combining the worlds of flavor and nutrition.

Evelyn has endured quite a while building this imaginative safe house. It's not only a cookbook; it's a zenith of her commitment to the craft of cooking and her enthusiasm for making feasts that are as really great for your spirit as they are for your taste buds. Every recipe is a part in her culinary excursion, reflecting long stretches of trial and error, refinement, and a pledge to making your time in the kitchen an upbeat experience.

What makes this excursion significantly more extraordinary? Evelyn's obligation to the weight reduction venture. She knows the battle, and these recipes are a demonstration of her devotion to making dinners that are delightful as well as aware of your wellbeing and health objectives.

It's not just about shedding pounds; it's tied in with embracing a way of life where nutritious decisions meet heavenly joys.

Anyway, what does the future hold for you? An excursion! Flip through these pages and let Evelyn guide you through a reality where flavors dance, surfaces play, and wellbeing cognizant enjoyments become the overwhelming focus. This cookbook contains more than just recipes; It's about embracing a way of life that combines health and good food.

Join Evelyn G. Powell on this culinary experience - where each dish is a festival, and the delight of cooking meets the way to a better, more delicious life.

TABLE OF CONTENTS

INTRODUCTION

Welcome to "Slim and Savory Diet cookbook 2024"! Setting out on an excursion towards a better way of life has never been more scrumptious and reachable. This cookbook is planned with you, the novice, as a main priority - somebody anxious to embrace the standards of the Weight Watchers program while getting a charge out of tasty and fulfilling feasts.

In these pages, you'll find an assortment of basic yet brilliant recipes, painstakingly created to make your culinary experience both pleasant and helpful. Each recipe is tailored to the SmartPoints system, giving you the support you need on your wellness journey, whether you're making a filling breakfast, a quick and delicious lunch, or a satisfying dinner. Not only that, but we also have mouthwatering recipes for soup, stew, fish and seafood. taking you on a culinary journey that consolidates the extravagance of the sea with the solace of a warm exquisite bowl. Drench yourself in the delicious kinds of our fish manifestations, painstakingly created to line up with the SmartPoints framework, guaranteeing a brilliant and irreproachable feasting experience.

Also, with regards to refreshments, our reviving solid choices are something other than drinks - they're dynamic blends intended to impeccably strengthen your faculties and supplement your dinners. Be that as it may, this cookbook goes past recipes. It's a manual for understanding the rudiments of the Weight Watchers program, settling on informed decisions while shopping for food, and continuously embracing a better relationship with food. You'll track down tips, stunts, and consolation to explore your direction through the universe of savvy and careful eating.

Thus, lock in, embrace the delectability, and how about we make 2024 your extended time of delicious change with "Slim and Savory Diet cookbook "

HOW TO USE THIS COOKBOOK

Welcome aboard! This cookbook is your compass for a flavorful journey towards a healthier you. Here's a quick guide on how to make the most of it.

1. First Date with the Introduction:
Start by giving the introduction a read. It's like meeting a new friend – get to know the cookbook's vibe and what it's all about.

2. Crack the SmartPoints Code: Don't be shy – embrace the SmartPoints section. It's like the secret language of this cookbook. Learn it, and you'll be a pro at making tasty meals with a healthy twist.

3. Chapters are Your GPS: Chapters are like different neighborhoods in this culinary city. Craving something specific? Navigate through the chapters to find the recipes that match your mood.

4. Plan Your Culinary Week: Use the book for meal planning. Pick recipes that suit your taste, mix them up, and plan meals for the week. Look for tips on prepping ahead to keep things stress-free.

5. Make It Yours: Don't follow recipes like strict rules. Feel free to swap ingredients or adjust portions. Make it your own culinary masterpiece – it's about enjoying the process as much as the meal.

6. Cooking Time is Adventure Time: Roll up your sleeves and get cooking. Each recipe comes with your cooking adventure guide – clear instructions, prep time, cook time, and serving sizes. Have fun in the kitchen!

7. Connect with the Community: Join the Weight Watchers crew. Share your kitchen triumphs, ask for advice, and connect with others on the same journey. It's like having a cooking buddy right in your pocket.

8. Cheers to Victories: Celebrate your wins. Mastered a new recipe? Hit a wellness goal? Celebrate! Every small victory counts, and this cookbook is here to cheer you on.

9. Beyond the Plate Wellness: Take a peek beyond the recipes. The book drops wisdom bombs on well-being outside the kitchen – from mindfulness to fitness. Little nuggets that can add some extra sparkle to your day.

10. Make It Your Culinary Playground: This book is like your culinary playground. Personalize it, scribble notes in the margins, and experiment. Let every recipe be a canvas for your wellness journey.

CHAPTER 1: **GETTING STARTED**

A Beginner's Guide To Grocery Shopping

When you stroll into a supermarket, do you continue onward with reason, knowing precisely everything you want and where to track it down? Or on the other hand do you feel questionable and befuddled, similar to you missing the example of the most proficient method to staple shop?

It tends to be enjoyable to browse among every one of the various brands and items, yet it's terrible to open your refrigerator or storeroom a couple of days after the fact and wish you had arranged your shopping trip somewhat better .Don't give up hope even if the thought of going grocery shopping makes you feel helpless! You can figure out how to staple shop like an ace in the blink of an eye with these convenient tips.

Instructions To Basic Food Item Shopping: Make an arrangement before you go. Beginning with a well-thought-out strategy is the first step in mastering grocery shopping. This will keep you from beginning overpowered, and provide you a substantial motivation when you enter the store.

Your arrangement ought to incorporate three essential parts: making a rundown of things you want, choosing where to shop, and arranging the best opportunity to shop.

The Most Effective Method To Make A Shopping List: A shopping list is your main protection system against the endeavors of the supermarket to part you from your cash.

This list is one that you will find very useful, even if you are not a big fan of lists. Unless you enjoy going to the store every other day to get something you forgot.) Therefore, how is a shopping list created?

Layouts Versus Free Form: Using a template as a starting point is one option. These rundown essential classes of food (dairy, meat/protein, produce) or even unambiguous food sources (milk, eggs, bread, apples). You should simply verify which things you want, and make a beeline for the store.

These templates are meant to make it easier for you to remember what you're out of. They can be useful on the off chance that you frequently wind up gazing into a for the most part void cooler considering what should be inside.

The downsides of utilizing layouts are that they are restricted to essential food varieties and fixings. Most layouts will have additional areas for you to write in things that aren't on the rundown, however assuming that you will quite often eat a variety of sorts of food sources, such records will not be extremely useful.

Attempting to find a format that rundowns the food varieties you consider rudiments could demonstrate a test, particularly in the event that you're on a unique eating regimen (in spite of the fact that I found an extremely careful veggie lover staple rundown, assuming you're into that). It's exhaustive to the point that I would have no desire to carry such a considerable rundown to the store with me!

Using a standard pen and paper, you can also create your own grocery list. I lean toward this choice since formats cause me to feel obliged in my food decisions.

PREPARE YOUR SHOPPING LIST

Whichever design you decide for your basic food item list, the initial step is to glance through your storeroom and fridge to see what you have and what you're out of.

Stand by, you say: how do I have any idea what I really want? Good query. Possibly you eat the very same food varieties consistently, or you make a dinner arrangement. Indeed, even an essential dinner plan will provide you with some thought of the fixings you'll require for the week.

Could you at any point go shopping for food without a dinner plan and staple rundown? Indeed, however it's simpler to wind up with food sources that don't go together or an excess of lettuce that you wind up tossing out when it spoils.Since it has become so undeniably obvious what food sources you really want, now is the ideal time to arrange your rundown.

ORGANIZE YOUR LIST BY DEPARTMENT OR AISLE: Contemplate which side of the store you ordinarily start at, and work your direction to the opposite side intellectually. Then record things in the request that you will pass them. This makes it simpler to recollect all that when you're in the store. For instance, I as a rule start in the dairy division, and end with produce (so it doesn't get crunched!).

On the off chance that you're new at this, you might have to record every one of the things you really want first, and afterward sort out the rundown on a different piece of paper. That is completely fine! You'll become acclimated to it rapidly.

PICK A PLACE TO SHOP

You could reside in a modest little town where there's just a single supermarket. Yet, chances are, you live within driving distance of a few different chain supermarkets, as well as different sorts of specialty stores or markets. In the event that you do, you want to settle on certain conclusions about where to shop.

Certain individuals like to purchase however much they can from their neighborhood rancher's market, and fill in different things at a characteristic food sources store. Others favor bigger chain stores since they can track down everything from apples to toothpaste in one spot.

Advantages of shopping at general stores: it's an all inclusive resource. On the off chance that you could do without running all over town, you can find essentially all that you really want here.

Likewise, these stores normally post deals pamphlets on the web and in nearby papers, and many have dependability programs which reward clients with gas limits or refunds.

Disadvantages of stores: the choice changes generally by store. Compared to bulk/wholesale stores, prices may be higher. It can be overwhelming to have so many options in one location, and you might end up spending more than you planned to.

THE BEST TIME TO SHOP

When is the best time to shop for groceries? Indeed, that relies a little upon your timetable and vicinity to the store.

At the point when you're simply figuring out how to staple shop, it could require an investment to conclude which time and day is best for you. However, the following are a couple of pointers to picking a great time.

What's the most exceedingly awful chance to go shopping for food? At the point when you're ravenous. I've committed this deadly error a few times, and consistently end up with pointless buys. The condition of your stomach is the main thing to consider while picking a chance to shop.

Then, think about your timetable and the external temperature. Assuming it's exceptionally hot or cold, plan your excursion with the goal that you can head home following shopping. Food varieties that should be kept virus ought to be refrigerated in something like two hours, or less assuming it's extremely hot outside. Consider bringing a cooler or cold bag with you when purchasing frozen foods during the summer.

In the colder time of year, freezing temperatures can harm fragile leafy foods, and cause surface changes in some dairy items. Something else to ponder is high traffic times in the store. There are in every case more individuals shopping at the end of the week, and late evening/evening is a more occupied time than morning. On the off chance that a jam-packed store makes you bound to fail to remember things, attempt to shop when the store isn't as occupied.

The fact that items are typically marked down in the morning is a final point. If you have any desire to find bargains on meat and dairy items, shopping prior is better.

Meal planning tips for beginners

Meal planning can be your kitchen's mystery ingredient for a smoother, more coordinated life. Here are a rational tips to cause meal planning wanting to feel less like an errand and more like a delicious experience:

- **Week by week Meeting:** Pick a day every week to design your feasts. Look at your calendar, think about busy days, and make plans accordingly. No requirement for an extravagant organizer - a straightforward schedule or note pad will do.

- **List Love:** Keep a running staple rundown of your priority things. It resembles a cheat sheet for your shopping experiences. It can be broken down by meals to make it easier to visit the store.

- **Flavor It Up:** Try not to allow your feasts to be a rerun. Varieties in grains, vegetables, and proteins keep things interesting. Attempt topic evenings for a fun loving turn.

- **Prep Like an Ace:** Cook once, eat two times. Batch cooking is a friend of yours. Prep fixings ahead of time for faster dinners during the week. Freeze additional items for those furious days.

- **Extra Lovin':** Plan for extras. Cook some extra, and presto - lunch for later is arranged. Be vital, putting heartier feasts prior in the week for simple reusing.

- **Desires Rule:** Be adaptable. Change things up if you're craving a particular dish. Desires are your body's approach to letting you know what it needs.

- **Tech-Accommodating Partners:** Give your phone a helping hand. Take a look at meal planning apps—they're like having a personal chef who gives you ideas for recipes, shopping lists, and some convenience.

- **Reflect and Rehash:** Pause for a minute toward the week's end to see what worked and what didn't. Change your arrangement as needs be. Commend your triumphs, huge or little - you're the expert of your kitchen space.

Meal planning is less about unbending principles and more about making life in the kitchen a touch more pleasant. With these tips, you're not simply arranging feasts; you're creating a menu for a more delicious, more coordinated way of life.

How to Make Meal Planning a Habit

To transform meal planning into a propensity, plan it into your daily practice. After you've achieved multi weeks of dinner arranging, you'll probably require another enormous shopping for food excursion or conveyance. Simply repeat the cycle and proceed with your daily practice until it turns out to be natural.

Following two or three weeks, you will probably see what is working for yourself and what isn't. Assuming you start straightforward in your most memorable little while, you can stretch out with additional involved or imaginative recipes, or even start to incorporate more dinners and snacks into your preparation and prep.

It's likewise astute to ensure you have all that you really want to make feast arranging and prep simple. You will need a sufficient number of food storage containers to store the foods you have prepared and cooked, in addition to any essentials you will keep in your fridge and cupboards. Different things to consider are feast arranging worksheets or records and names for your dinners or feast arranging applications that can make the interaction more straightforward.

CHAPTER 2: **BREAKFAST BOOSTERS**

<u>Healthy Oatmeal Pancakes</u>

Prep time:
10 mins
Cook time:15 mins
Servings:4
SmartPoints:4

INGREDIENTS
- 1 1⁄2 cups skim milk

- 1⁄4 cup canola oil

- 1 egg

- 2 egg whites

- 3⁄4 cup white flour

- 3⁄4 cup whole wheat flour

- 1⁄2 cup oatmeal

- 1 tablespoon baking

powder

- 1⁄2 teaspoon allspice or
  1/2 teaspoon cinnamon

- 1⁄4 teaspoon salt

DIRECTIONS

1. Heat an electric frypan or pancake griddle, lightly oiling it with nonstick cooking spray.

2. Whisk together the milk, oil, and eggs (wet ingredients); then, combine the other (dry) ingredients and add them to the wet ingredients; whisk to blend everything.

3. Pour 1/4 cup of batter at a time onto a hot griddle to form 5-6" pancakes; cook until the surface of the pancakes is bubbled; flip pancakes over and cook until both sides are light golden brown.

NOTES: The proportion of white flour to entire wheat flour can undoubtedly be fluctuated (model: 1 cup white flour and 1/2 cup wheat flour) to suit the preferences of your family. You can likewise skirt the egg whites and utilize two whole eggs. Also, for this recipe, your decision of either speedy cooking or customary designed cereal will turn out great.

Nutrition Facts
(per serving)
400 calories
50g carbs
14g Protein
16g Fat

Spinach And Egg Scramble With Raspberries

Prep Time: 10 mins
Servings:1
SmartPoints: 1

Ingredients

- 1 teaspoon canola oil

- 1 ½ cups baby spinach (1 1/2 ounces)

- 2 large eggs, lightly beaten

- Pinch of kosher salt

- Pinch of ground pepper

- 1 slice whole-grain bread, toasted

- ½ cup fresh raspberries

Directions

1. In a small nonstick skillet set over medium-high heat, heat the oil. Stir the spinach often and simmer for one to two minutes, or until it wilts. Turn the spinach onto a platter. Add the eggs, cover the pan, and heat it at a medium temperature. For even cooking, toss once or twice while cooking. Cook for one to two minutes, or until just set. Add the

salt, pepper, and spinach and stir. Along with bread and strawberries, serve the scramble.

Nutrition Facts
(per serving)
Calories: 296
Fat: 16g
Carbs: 21g
Protein: 18g

Peanut Butter And Chia Berry Jam English Muffin

Cook Time: 10 mins
Servings:1
SmartPoints:1

Ingredients

- ½ cup unsweetened mixed frozen berries

- 2 teaspoons chia seeds

- 2 teaspoons natural peanut butter

- 1 whole-wheat English muffin, toasted

Directions

1. Microwave berries in a medium microwave-safe bowl for 30 seconds; mix and microwave 30 seconds more. Mix in chia seeds.

2. Spread peanut butter on the English muffin. Top with the berry-chia mixture.

Nutrition Facts
(per serving)
262 Calories
9g Fat
41g Carbs
10g Protein

Strawberry-Ricotta Waffle Sandwich

Prep Time: 10 mins
Servings:1
SmartPoints:1

Ingredients

- ¼ cup whole-milk ricotta cheese

- 1 teaspoon chopped fresh mint or basil

- ½ teaspoon vanilla extract

- 2 frozen whole-grain waffles, toasted (see Tips)

- 2 teaspoons pure maple syrup

- ½ cup sliced fresh strawberries

Directions

- In a small bowl, combine ricotta, mint (or basil), and vanilla. Drizzle each waffle with 1 teaspoon syrup. Top one waffle with the ricotta mixture and strawberries, then cover with the second waffle.

Tips: To choose a healthy frozen waffle, check for whole grains mentioned first (after water) in the ingredient list and at least 3 grams of fiber per 2-waffle serving. Choose ones with 200 or fewer calories, 4 grams of sugar, and 350 mg of salt per 2 waffles.

Nutrition Facts
(per serving)
318 Calories
14g Fat
43g Carbs
12g Protein

Blueberry-Ricotta Pancakes

Cook Time: 40 mins
Servings:4
SmartPoints:1

Ingredients
- 1/2 cup whole-wheat pastry flour (see Source)

- 1/4 cup plus 2 tablespoons all-purpose flour

- 1 teaspoon sugar

- 1 teaspoon baking powder

- ¼ teaspoon baking soda

- ½ teaspoon freshly grated nutmeg

- ¾ cup part-skim ricotta cheese

- 1 large egg

- 1 large egg white

- 1/2 cup nonfat buttermilk (see Tip)

- 1 teaspoon freshly grated lemon zest

- 1 tablespoon lemon juice

- 2 teaspoons canola oil, divided

- ¾ cup fresh or frozen (not thawed) blueberries

Directions

1. Whisk entire wheat flour, regular flour, sugar, baking powder, baking pop and nutmeg in a little bowl. Whisk ricotta, egg, egg white, buttermilk, lemon zing and juice in a huge bowl until smooth. Gently combine the wet and dry components.

2. Brush an enormous nonstick skillet with 1/2 teaspoon oil and spot over medium intensity until hot. Utilizing a liberal 1/4 cup of player for every hotcake, pour the batter for 2 flapjacks into the skillet, sprinkle blueberries on every flapjack and cook until the edges are dry and air pockets start to frame, around 2 minutes. Flip the flapjacks and cook until brilliant brown, around 2 minutes more. Rehash with the leftover oil, hitter and berries, changing the intensity as important to forestall consuming.

Nutrition Facts
(per serving)
237 Calories
8g Fat
30g Carbs
12g Protein

<u>**Waffles**</u>

Cook Time: 40 mins
Servings:6

Ingredients
- 1 cup whole-wheat flour

- 1 cup all-purpose flour

- 1 ½ teaspoons baking powder

- ½ teaspoon salt

- ¼ teaspoon baking soda

- 2 cups nonfat buttermilk, (see Tip)

- 1 large egg, separated

- 1 tablespoon canola oil

- 1 tablespoon vanilla extract, (optional)

- 2 large egg whites

- 2 tablespoons sugar

Directions

1. In a large mixing bowl, add whole wheat flour, all-purpose flour, baking powder, salt, and baking soda. Whisk buttermilk, the egg yolk, oil and vanilla (if utilizing) in a different bowl. Add the wet fixings to the dry fixings and mix with a wooden spoon just until dampened.

2. Beat the 3 egg whites in an oil free blending bowl with an electric blender until delicate pinnacles structure. Add sugar and keep beating until firm and lustrous. Whisk one-fourth of the beaten egg whites into the player. Using a rubber spatula, fold in the remaining beaten egg whites.

3. Preheat a waffle iron. Use oil to lightly brush the surface. Fill the waffle iron 66% brimming with a player. Cook until the waffles are fresh and brilliant, 5 to 6 minutes. Rehash with the excess hitter, brushing the surface with oil prior to cooking each group.

Nutrition Facts
(per serving)
229 Calories
4g Fat
39g Carbs
10g Protein

Banana-Cocoa Soy Smoothie

Cook Time: 5 mins
Servings:1
SmartPoints: 1

Ingredients
- 1 banana

- ½ cup silken tofu

- ½ cup soymilk

- 2 tablespoons unsweetened cocoa powder

- 1 tablespoon honey

Directions
1. Cut banana and freeze until firm. Mix tofu, soymilk, cocoa and honey in a blender until smooth. With the engine running, add the banana cuts through the opening in the top and keep on pureeing until smooth.

Nutrition Facts
(per serving)
342 Calories
8g Fat
62g Carbs
16g Protein

Salad With Quinoa And Strawberries

Cook Time: 15 mins
Servings: 1
SmartPoints:1

Ingredients

- 1 teaspoon minced garlic

- Pinch of salt

- 1 tablespoon extra-virgin olive oil

- 2 teaspoons red-wine vinegar

- Pinch of ground pepper

- 3 cups lightly packed baby kale

- ½ cup cooked quinoa

- ½ cup sliced strawberries

- 1 tablespoon salted pepitas

Directions

1. Make a paste by combining the salt and garlic with the side of a chef's knife or fork. Whisk the garlic glue, oil, vinegar and pepper together in a medium bowl. Include kale toss for a coat. Top with strawberries, quinoa, and pepitas.

Nutrition Facts

(per serving)
330 Calories
20g Fat
31g Carbs
9g Protein

CHAPTER 3: SNACKS AND APPETIZER DELIGHTS

Blue Cheese And Pear Tartlets

Prep Time:10 mins
Cook Time:15 mins
Servings:15

IIngredient
- ripe pear - peeled, cored, and chopped

- 4 ounces blue cheese, crumbled

- 2 tablespoons light cream

- ground black pepper to taste

- 1 (1.9 ounce) package mini phyllo tart shells

Directions
1. Heat the stove to 350 degrees F (175 degrees C).

2. Combine as one pear, blue cheddar, and cream in a baking dish. Use pepper to season. Spoon combination into phyllo shells.

3. Prepare in the preheated stove for 15 minutes. Keep warm.

Nutrition Facts
(per serving)
60 Calories
4g Fat
5g Carbs
2g Protein

<u>Christmas Dip</u>

Prep Time: 20 mins
Additional Time: 2 hrs
Servings: 24
Yield: 4 cups

Ingredients

- 1 (6 ounce) package dried cranberries

- 1 cup chopped pistachio nuts

- 1 (8 ounce) package cream cheese, softened

- ½ cup butter, softened

- 2 ounces crumbled blue cheese

- 4 ounces Brie cheese, rind removed

Directions

1. For garnish, reserve 1 tablespoon each of dried cranberries and pistachios. Join the remaining dried cranberries and pistachio nuts in a little bowl. Line a little round blending bowl in with saran wrap.

2. Beat together cream cheddar, margarine, blue cheddar, and Brie in a bowl until smooth. Spread 1/3 of the cheddar combination equitably in the lower part of the cling wrap-lined bowl. Layer 1/3 of the cranberry-nut combination over the cheddar. Layer cheddar blend

with berry-nut combination two times more, finishing with a layer of cranberry-pistachio combination.

3. Cover the bowl with more wrap, squeezing the wrap down onto the spread to pack it. Refrigerate for a few hours or short-term. To serve, take plastic wrap off the highest point of the bowl and turn the layered plunge out onto a serving dish. Eliminate staying plastic wrap, and sprinkle held cranberries and pistachios around the spread to embellish.

Note:
Present with fresh Moravian-style zest treats or gingersnaps for a fiery differentiation of flavors.

Nutrition Facts
(per serving)
142 Calories
12g Fat
8g Carbs
3g Protein

Puff Pastry Christmas Tree

Prep Time:35 mins
Cook Time:20 mins
Servings:8
Yield:8 servings

Ingredients

- 2 tablespoons sun-dried tomato pesto

- 2 tablespoons soft goat cheese

- 2 sheets puff pastry

- 2 tablespoons freshly grated Pecorino-Romano cheese, divided

- 1 egg, beaten

- ½ teaspoon dried oregano

Directions

1. Heat the stove to 400 degrees F (200 degrees C). Use parchment paper to line a baking sheet.

2. Join sun-dried tomato pesto and goat cheddar in a little bowl and mix well.

3. Unroll 1 puff cake sheet onto the pre-arranged baking sheet. Remove 2 strips at the lower part of the sheet to shape a tree trunk, around 1 inch wide and tall. Slice slantingly to the highest point of the puff

cake sheet to make a long three-sided shape, eliminating overabundant baked goods on one or the other side.

4. Spread a far layer of the pesto combination over the baked good, the whole way to the sides. Sprinkle 1 tablespoon Pecorino-Romano cheddar on top.

5. Roll up the second puff cake sheet and spot at the tip of the triangle. Unroll cautiously towards the base. To match the first triangle, lightly press down and cut away the sides with care. Eliminate overabundant cake.

6. From the trunk to the tip, cut branches that are 1/3 of an inch thick into the sides of the triangle from both sides, leaving a space in the middle that runs lengthwise. Wind the branches from you, attempting to get in 2 turns on the lower branches. Keep climbing the tree, contorting away from you as you go.

7. Brush the whole tree with beaten egg. Sprinkle 1 tablespoon of Pecorino-Romano cheddar and dried oregano.

8. Bake for about 20 minutes in a preheated oven until a deep golden brown. Allow to slightly cool on the baking sheet.

Notes:

You can substitute cream cheese for spreadable goat cheese. You can also substitute basil pesto for sun-dried tomato pesto or spread.

If desired, cut a star out of the excess pastry and lay it on top of the tree, then brush with egg.

Nutrition Facts
(per serving)
355 Calories
25g Fat
28g Carbs
6g Protein

<u>Sausage Balls</u>

Prep Time:10 mins
Cook Time:20 mins
Servings:15
Yield:30 sausage balls

Ingredients

- 1 pound ground pork sausage, at room temperature

- 2 cups biscuit baking mix

- 1 pound sharp Cheddar cheese, shredded

- Sausage: This sausage balls recipe starts with a pound of ground pork sausage. Use hot ground sausage for a spicy kick.

- Baking mix: Use a store-bought mix, such as Bisquick, or make your own at home with pantry staples.

- Cheese: These sausage balls wouldn't be complete without shredded Cheddar.

Directions

1. Heat the stove to 350 degrees F (175 degrees C).

2. Consolidate room temperature wiener and roll blend in an enormous bowl; blend in with your hands until very much joined. Add destroyed cheddar and blend until completely integrated. Fold into around 30 pecan estimated balls; move to a baking sheet.

Nutrition Facts
(per serving)
264 Calories
19g Fat
11g Carbs
13g Protein

<u>**Lemon-Garlic Marinated Shrimp**</u>

Active Time:10 mins
Servings:12
SmartPoints:12
Ingredients
- 3 tablespoons minced garlic

- 2 tablespoons extra-virgin olive oil

- ¼ cup lemon juice

- ¼ cup minced fresh parsley

- ½ teaspoon kosher salt

- ½ teaspoon pepper

- 1 ¼ pounds cooked shrimp

Directions
Place garlic and oil in a little skillet and cook over medium intensity until fragrant, around 1 moment. Add lemon juice, parsley, salt and pepper. Throw with shrimp in an enormous bowl. Chill until prepared to serve.

Nutrition Facts
(per serving)
82 Calories
3g Fat
2g Carbs
11g Protein

Marshmallow Fruit Dip

Prep time: 10 min
SmartPoints: 5 cups (40 servings)

Ingredients
- 1 package (8 ounces) cream cheese, softened

- 3/4 cup cherry yogurt

- 1 carton (8 ounces) frozen whipped topping, thawed

- 1 jar (7 ounces) marshmallow creme

- Assorted fresh fruit

Directions
In an enormous bowl, beat cream cheese and yogurt until mixed. Overlap in whipped garnish and marshmallow creme. Present with organic products.

Nutrition Facts
2 tablespoons:
56 calories
3g fat (2g saturated fat)
7 mg cholesterol
24mg sodium
6g carbohydrate (5g sugars, 0 fiber),
1g protein.

<u>**Sushi Rolls**</u>

Prep: 1 hour
Makes: 64 pieces

Ingredients
- 2 cups sushi rice, rinsed and drained

- 2 cups water

- 1/4 cup rice vinegar

- 2 tablespoons sugar

- 1/2 teaspoon salt

- 2 tablespoons sesame seeds, toasted

- 2 tablespoons black sesame seeds

- Bamboo sushi mat

- 8 nori sheets

- 1 small cucumber, seeded and julienned

- 3 ounces imitation crab meat sticks, julienned

- 1 medium ripe avocado, peeled and julienned

- Optional: Reduced-sodium soy sauce, prepared wasabi and pickled ginger slices

Directions

1. Combine the rice and water in a large saucepan; allow to sit for 30 minutes. Heat to the point of boiling. Turn heat down to low; cover and stew for 15-20 minutes or until water is assimilated and rice is delicate. Eliminate from the intensity. Let stand, covered, for 10 minutes.

2. In the meantime, in a little bowl, join the vinegar, sugar and salt, mixing until sugar is disintegrated.

3. Place the rice in a big, shallow bowl; use the vinegar mixture to drizzle. To slightly cool the rice, stir it with a wooden paddle or spoon in a slicing motion. Cover with a sodden fabric to keep wet. (Rice combination might be made as long as 2 hours ahead and put away at room temperature, covered with a clammy towel. Refrigerate not.)

4. Sprinkle toasted and dark sesame seeds onto a plate; put away. Put the sushi mat on a work surface so the mat rolls from you; line with saran wrap. Place 3/4 cup rice on plastic. Rice should be pressed into an 8-inch square. Add one nori sheet on top.

5. Organize a modest quantity of cucumber, crab and avocado around 1-1/2 in. from the base edge of the nori sheet. Turn up rice blend over filling, utilizing the bamboo mat to lift and pack the combination while rolling; eliminate plastic wrap as you roll.

6. Eliminate mat; roll sushi rolls in sesame seeds. Cover with cling wrap. Rehash with outstanding fixings to make 8 rolls. Cut each into 8 pieces. Present with soy sauce, wasabi and ginger cuts whenever wanted.

Nutrition Facts
1 piece:
35 calories,
1g fat (0 saturated fat)
0 cholesterol
30mg sodium
6g carbohydrate (1g sugars, 1g fiber)
1g protein
Diabetic Exchanges: 1/2 starch

Cherry Tomato Bites

Prep time: 30 min
SmartPoints: about 4 dozen

Ingredients

- 2 pints cherry tomatoes

- 1 package (8 ounces) cream cheese, softened

- 6 bacon strips, cooked and crumbled

- 1/4 cup finely chopped green onions

- 1/4 cup minced fresh parsley

- 1/4 teaspoon Worcestershire sauce

Directions

Remove a flimsy cut the highest point of every tomato. Scoop out and dispose of mash. Rearrange the tomatoes on a paper towel to deplete. In the meantime, join remaining fixings in a little bowl. Spoon into tomatoes. Refrigerate until serving.

Nutrition Facts

3 each:
72 calories
6g fat (4g saturated fat)
18mg cholesterol
85 mg sodium

2g carbohydrate (1g sugars, 0 fiber)
2g protein

CHAPTER 4: **LUNCH ON THE GO**

Veggie And Hummus Sandwich

Time: 10 mins
Servings:1
SmartPoints:1

Ingredients

- 2 slices whole-grain bread

- 3 tablespoons hummus

- ¼ avocado, mashed

- ½ cup mixed salad greens

- ¼ medium red bell pepper, sliced

- ¼ cup sliced cucumber

- ¼ cup shredded carrot

Directions

Spread 1 cut of bread with hummus and the other with avocado. Add cucumber, carrot, ringer pepper, and greens to the sandwich. Cut fifty and serve.

Nutrition Facts
(per serving)
325 Calories
14g Fat
40g Carbs
13g Protein

Buffalo Chicken Grain Bowl

Prep Time: 10 mins
Servings:1
SmartPoints: 4

Ingredients

- ⅔ cup cooked whole-wheat couscous (see associated recipe)

- 2 tablespoons honey-mustard vinaigrette, divided (see associated recipe)

- 1 roasted chicken thigh, sliced (see associated recipe)

- 2 stalks celery, chopped

- 1 carrot, peeled and cut into ribbons with a vegetable peeler

- 2 tablespoons crumbled blue cheese

- Hot sauce to taste

Directions

In a medium container with a seal, combine the couscous and one tablespoon of dressing. Top with chicken, celery, carrot strips and blue cheddar. Apply the remaining 1 tablespoon of dressing to the dish. Refrigerate for as long as 5 days. Top with hot sauce not long prior to serving.

Nutrition Facts

(per serving)
579 Calories

32g Fat
42g Carbs
32g Protein

Chickpea Chicken Salad

Prep Time: 10 mins
Servings:4
SmartPoints: 4

Ingredients

- ½ cup canola mayonnaise

- 3 tablespoons chopped fresh flat-leaf parsley

- 2 tablespoons chopped fresh dill

- 1 ½ teaspoons country-style Dijon mustard

- ½ teaspoon kosher salt

- ½ teaspoon smoked paprika

- ¼ teaspoon ground pepper

- 2 (15 ounce) cans no-salt-added chickpeas, rinsed

- ½ cup chopped celery (from 2 stalks)

- ¼ cup finely chopped shallot (from 1 large shallot)

Directions

Join mayonnaise, parsley, dill, mustard, salt, paprika and pepper in a bowl. Add chickpeas, celery and shallot; mix until very much covered.

Tips:
To make ahead: Refrigerate in a water/air proof compartment for as long as 4 days.

Nutrition Facts
(per serving)
300 Calories
9g Fat
37g Carbs
12g Protein

Sesame Instant Ramen Noodles with Broccoli And Soft-Boiled Egg

Prep Time: 10 mins
Servings:1
SmartPoints: 2

Ingredients

- 3 cups water

- 1 cup frozen broccoli

- 1 (3 ounce) package ramen-noodle soup mix

- 1 teaspoon toasted sesame oil

- ½ teaspoon toasted sesame seeds

- 1 large soft-boiled egg, halved (see Tip)

Directions

1. Carry water to bubble in a medium pan. Add broccoli; cook for 2 minutes. Noodles; save the seasoning packet for later; cook until the noodles are delicate, around 3 minutes more. Channel the broccoli and noodles and return to the container.

2. Add sesame oil, sesame seeds and a big part of the flavoring bundle (dispose of the rest of save for another utilization); throw well to consolidate. Move to a bowl; top with egg and serve.

Tips:

To delicate bubble eggs: Place eggs in a pan; add water to simply cover the eggs. Bring to a stew over medium-high intensity. Eliminate from intensity and let 2 to 3 minutes for amazing delicate set yolks.

Nutrition Facts

(per serving)

257 Calories

12g Fat

27g Carbs

14g Protein

Ham And Broccoli Topped Baked Potato

Prep Time: 10 mins
Servings:1
SmartPoints:1

Ingredients

- ½ cup small broccoli florets

- 3 tablespoons diced lower-sodium ham

- 1 6-ounce russet potato, baked

- 1 tablespoon plain nonfat Greek yogurt

- ¼ cup finely shredded reduced-fat Cheddar cheese

Directions

Cook the broccoli in a small microwave-safe bowl until just tender. Heat diced ham. Top potato with ham, broccoli, yogurt, and cheese.

Nutrition Facts
(per serving)
298 Calories
7g Fat
41g Carbs
19g Protein

<u>**Avocado Egg Salad**</u>

Prep Time: 10 mins
Servings:4
SmartPoints: 4

Ingredients

- 6 hard-boiled eggs, coarsely chopped

- 1 medium avocado

- 2 tablespoons lemon juice

- 1 tablespoon mayonnaise

- ½ teaspoon salt

- ¼ teaspoon ground pepper

- ⅓ cup finely chopped celery

- 2 tablespoons chopped fresh chives, plus more for garnish

Dircctions

Squash eggs, avocado, lemon juice, mayonnaise, salt and pepper together in a medium bowl until coarsely pounded and velvety. Crease in celery and chives. Embellish with extra chives, whenever wanted.

Nutrition Facts
(per serving)
224 Calories
18g Fat
6g Carbs
11g Protein

Tomato Soup With Beans And Greens

Prep Time:10 mins
Servings:4
SmartPoints: 4

Ingredients

- 2 (14 ounce) cans low-sodium hearty-style tomato soup

- 1 tablespoon olive oil

- 3 cups chopped kale

- 1 teaspoon minced garlic

- ⅛ teaspoon crushed red pepper (Optional)

- 1 (14 ounce) can no-salt-added cannellini beans, rinsed

- ¼ cup grated Parmesan cheese

Directions

1. Heat soup in a medium pot as per bundle headings; stew over low intensity as you plan kale.

2. Heat oil in an enormous skillet over medium intensity. Add kale and cook, blending, until withered, 1 to 2 minutes. Mix in garlic and crushed red pepper (if utilizing) and cook for 30 seconds. Mix the greens and beans into the soup and stew until the beans are warmed through, 2 to 3 minutes.

3.   Split the soup between 4 dishes. Serve finished off with Parmesan.

Nutrition Facts
(per serving)
200 Calories
6g Fat
29g Carbs
9g Protein

Chicken And Cabbage Bowls With Sesame Dressing

Time:10 mins
Servings: 4
SmartPoints:4

Ingredients

- 1 (12-ounce) package seasoned cooked chicken strips

- 1 (9-ounce) package shredded coleslaw mix

- 1/2 cup
  sesame-honey-flavored almonds

- 1/2 cup light sesame dressing

Directions

Cut chicken tenders into scaled down pieces. Partition coleslaw blend among 4 dishes. Top with the chicken and almonds. Sprinkle with dressing.

Nutrition information

Serving Size: 3/4 cup cabbage, 3 oz. chicken, 2 Tbsp. almonds and 2 Tbsp. dressing

Nutrition Facts

Calories 324,
Fat 21g (Saturated Fat 4g) Cholesterol 55 mg Carbohydrates 14g
Total Sugars 10g Added Sugars 8g
Protein 23g
Fiber 2g

Sodium 370mg
Potassium 116

CHAPTER 5: **DINNER MADE EASY**

<u>Wild Rice Stuffing with Apple & Sausage</u>

Cook Time:1 hr 15 mins
Additional Time:50 mins
Servings:14
Yield:14 servings, 1 cup each

Ingredients

- 1 ¼ cups wild rice (8 ounces)

- 4 cups cubed Jewish rye bread (1/2-inch cubes), preferably day-old

- 1 pound sweet turkey sausage, casings removed

- 2 cups chopped leeks, white and light green parts only

- 2 tart apples, cut into 1/4-inch dice

- 1 cup diced celery

- 3 cups reduced-sodium chicken or turkey broth

- 1 cup dried cherries

- 1 cup coarsely chopped pecans

- 1 ½ tablespoons minced fresh marjoram

- 2 teaspoons minced fresh thyme

- ¼ teaspoon salt

- ¼ teaspoon freshly ground pepper

Directions

1. Place the rice in a medium saucepan and add enough water to cover it by about 1 1/2 inches. Preheat the oven to 300 degrees F. Heat to the point of boiling. Diminish intensity to keep a stew, cover and cook until delicate, around 60 minutes. (Or on the other hand get ready as per bundle bearings.) Channel well.

2. Spread bread out on a baking sheet in the meantime; heat, blending once partially through, until dry and fresh, around 25 minutes.

3. Increment stove temperature to 425 degrees . Cover a 3-to 4-quart baking dish with cooking splash.

4. Around 15 minutes before the rice is finished, cook wiener and leeks in a huge skillet over medium intensity, blending and parting ways with a spoon, until the frankfurter is caramelized, 6 to 8 minutes. Cook for a further three minutes after adding the apples and celery.

5. In a large bowl, transfer the sausage mixture. Add the rice and bread, then mix in stock, cherries, walnuts, marjoram, thyme, salt and pepper. Move to the pre-arranged baking dish and cover firmly with foil.

6. Stuffing should be baked for 35 minutes. Uncover and heat until the top is cooked, 15 to 20 minutes more.

Nutrition Facts
(per serving)
291 Calories
9g Fat
40g Carbs
13g Protein

Carrot Casserole

Active Time:20 mins
Total Time:1 hr
Servings: 6 servings

Ingredients

- 5 medium carrots, peeled and thinly sliced (about 4 cups)

- 1 teaspoon water

- 1 teaspoon extra-virgin olive oil

- 1/2 cup whole-wheat panko breadcrumbs

- 2 teaspoons finely chopped fresh thyme

- 2 teaspoons finely chopped fresh flat-leaf parsley

- 1/4 teaspoon salt, divided
- 2 tablespoons unsalted butter

- 2 tablespoons all-purpose flour

- 1 1/2 cups whole milk

- 1 1/4 teaspoons dry mustard

- 1/2 teaspoon onion powder

- 1/4 teaspoon ground pepper

- 1/8 teaspoon ground coriander

- 1 cup shredded Cheddar cheese, divided

Directions

1. Preheat the oven to 375°F. Cooking spray a 9-by-6-inch baking dish lightly. Place carrots and water in an enormous microwaveable bowl. Cover with cling wrap; microwave on High until fresh delicate, 4 to 5 minutes.

2. Heat oil in a huge skillet over medium-high intensity. 1/8 teaspoon salt, thyme, parsley, and panko cook, mixing periodically, until the panko is brilliant brown, around 3 minutes. Place the ingredients in a small bowl. Clean the skillet off.

3. Soften spread in the skillet over medium intensity. Race in flour. Cook, whisking continually, for 1 moment. Progressively speed in milk until a smooth and somewhat thickened sauce structures, around 1 moment. Add mustard, onion powder, pepper and coriander. Cook, blending periodically, until the sauce thickens, around 4 minutes. Eliminate from heat.

4. Put half of the sauce in the baking dish that has been prepared. Add half of the carrots; top with 1/2 cup Cheddar. Use the remaining sauce, carrots, and Cheddar in a similar manner. Sprinkle the remaining 1/8 teaspoon of salt on top before covering with the panko mixture. Cover with foil.

5. Prepare for 25 minutes. Remove the cover and bake for about 10 minutes, or until the carrots are tender and the sauce is bubbling. Let cool for 5 minutes prior to serving.

Nutrition Facts
(per serving)
218 Calories
14g Fat
16g Carbs
8g Protein

Baked Mac And Cheese

Cook Time:25 mins
Additional Time:30 mins
Servings:4
Yield:4 servings

Ingredients

- 3 tablespoons plain dry breadcrumbs, (see Tip)

- 1 teaspoon extra-virgin olive oil

- ¼ teaspoon paprika

- 1 16-ounce or 10-ounce package frozen spinach, thawed

- 1 ¾ cups low-fat milk, divided

- 3 tablespoons all-purpose flour

- 2 cups shredded extra-sharp Cheddar cheese

- 1 cup low-fat cottage cheese

- ⅛ teaspoon ground nutmeg

- ¼ teaspoon salt

- Freshly ground pepper, to taste

- 8 ounces (2 cups) whole-wheat elbow macaroni, or penne

Directions

1. Preheat the oven to 375°F. Cooking spray a 9-by-6-inch baking dish lightly. Place carrots and water in an enormous microwaveable bowl. Cover with cling wrap; microwave on High until fresh delicate, 4 to 5 minutes.

2. Heat oil in a huge skillet over medium-high intensity. 1/8 teaspoon salt, thyme, parsley, and panko cook, mixing periodically, until the panko is brilliant brown, around 3 minutes. Place the ingredients in a small bowl. Clean the skillet off.

3. Soften spread in the skillet over medium intensity. Race in flour. Cook, whisking continually, for 1 moment. Progressively speed in milk until a smooth and somewhat thickened sauce structures, around 1 moment. Add mustard, onion powder, pepper and coriander. Cook, blending periodically, until the sauce thickens, around 4 minutes. Eliminate from heat.

4. Put half of the sauce in the baking dish that has been prepared. Add half of the carrots; top with 1/2 cup Cheddar. Use the remaining sauce, carrots, and Cheddar in a similar manner. Sprinkle the remaining 1/8 teaspoon of salt on top before covering with the panko mixture. Cover with foil.

5. Prepare for 25 minutes. Remove the cover and bake for about 10 minutes, or until the carrots are tender and the sauce is bubbling. Let cool for 5 minutes prior to serving.

Nutrition Facts
(per serving)
584 Calories
24g Fat
60g Carbs
38g Protein

Chicken Noodle Soup With Spinach And Parmesan Cheese

Active Time:15 mins
Total Time:20 mins
Servings: 4 servings

Ingredients

- 2 tablespoons extra-virgin olive oil

- 2 cloves garlic, thinly sliced

- 1/4 teaspoon crushed red pepper

- 1/3 cup dry white wine

- 6 cups low-sodium chicken broth

- 1/4 teaspoon salt

- 1/4 teaspoon ground pepper

- 1/2 cup whole-wheat small elbow pasta

- 2 cups shredded cooked chicken breast

- 1 (5 ounce) package baby spinach

- 1/2 teaspoon lemon zest

- 2 tablespoons lemon juice

- 1/3 cup finely grated Parmesan cheese

Directions

1. Cook oil, garlic and crushed red pepper in a medium pan over medium-high intensity, mixing continually, until fragrant and sizzling, around 2 minutes. Mix in wine; cook, blending once, until diminished significantly, around 2 minutes.

2. Take off the heat. Add chicken and spinach; mix until the spinach is withered, around 1 moment. Mix in lemon zing and lemon juice.

3. Split the soup between 4 shallow dishes; sprinkle with Parmesan cheese.

Nutrition facts
Serving Size: 1 3/4 cups
Calories 277
Fat 11g,
Saturated Fat 3g
Cholesterol 53 mg Carbohydrates 16g, Total Sugars 2g, Added Sugars 0g,
Protein 25g,
Fiber 2g,
Sodium 544mg,
Potassium 222mg

Noodle Soup With Buttery Tomato Broth

Active Time:10 mins
Total Time:20 mins
Servings: 4 servings

Ingredients

- 1 tablespoon canola oil

- 1 tablespoon garlic paste

- 1 tablespoon ginger paste

- 1/4 cup unsalted tomato paste

- 4 cups reduced-sodium chicken broth

- 1 (3-inch) cinnamon stick

- 3 whole star anise

- 1 teaspoon black peppercorns

- 4 tablespoons unsalted butter, cut into pieces

- 2 teaspoons fish sauce

- 9 ounces fresh udon noodles

- 4 teaspoons toasted sesame oil

- 1/4 cup thinly sliced scallions

- 1 teaspoon toasted white or black sesame seeds

Directions

1. In a medium saucepan, heat canola oil to a medium-high temperature. Add garlic glue and ginger glue; cook, mixing continually, until fragrant, around 1 moment. Utilize tomato paste; cook, mixing continually, until marginally obscured, around 1 moment. Add the broth, cinnamon stick, peppercorns, and star anise; cover and heat to the point of boiling over high intensity. Decrease intensity to medium to keep a stew; stew for 10 minutes. Mix in margarine and fish sauce, racing to totally soften the spread.

2. In the meantime, heat a huge pot of water to the point of boiling. Noodles should be cooked as directed on the package. Drain.

3. Split the noodles between 4 shallow dishes. Scoop 1 cup of the stock over each; shower each bowl with 1 teaspoon sesame oil. Sprinkle with scallions and sesame seeds.

Nutrition Facts
Serving Size: 1 3/4 cups
Calories 322
Fat 22g(Saturated Fat 8g)
Cholesterol 31 mg Carbohydrates 27g
Total Sugars 4g, Added Sugars 0g,
Protein 5g
Fiber 1g
Sodium 681mg
Potassium 202 mg

Smoked Turkey, Kale And Rice Bake

Active Time: 20 mins
Additional Time: 20 mins
Total Time:40 mins
Servings:6
Yield:6 servings, about 1 1/3 cups each

Ingredients

- 1 tablespoon extra-virgin olive oil

- 2 cups thinly sliced leeks, white and light green parts only

- 1 cup thinly sliced celery

- 4 cups slivered kale leaves

- 1 28-ounce can diced tomatoes

- 1 cup low-fat, no-salt-added cottage cheese

- 1 cup instant or quick-cooking brown rice

- 6 ounces smoked turkey breast or smoked tofu, chopped (1 1/2 cups)

- ¼ cup water

- 1 teaspoon freshly ground pepper, or to taste

- 1 cup shredded extra-sharp Cheddar cheese

Directions

1. Over medium-high heat, heat oil in a large, broiler-safe skillet. Cook the celery and leeks for 2 to 3 minutes, stirring frequently, until they begin to soften.

2. Add kale and tomatoes and cook, blending, until the kale starts to shrink, 1 to 2 minutes. Mix in curds, rice, turkey (or tofu), water and pepper. Bring to a stew. Diminish intensity to medium-low, cover and cook for 10 minutes.

3. Set the rack in the upper third of the oven while this is going on; preheat the oven.

4. Increase the heat to medium, stir the rice mixture, and cook, uncovered, for 10 to 12 minutes or until most of the liquid has evaporated. Spread cheddar on top. Cook until the cheddar is foaming, 2 to 3 minutes.

Nutrition Facts

(per serving)
266 Calories
11g Fat
26g Carbs
18g Protein

Creamy Lemon-Basil Chicken

Active Time:20 mins
Total Time:20 mins
Servings:4

Ingredients

- 1 pound chicken cutlets (4 cutlets)

- ½ teaspoon salt

- ½ teaspoon ground pepper

- 2 tablespoons unsalted butter, divided

- 2 teaspoons minced garlic

- 1 ¼ cups unsalted chicken broth

- 3 ounces reduced-fat cream cheese, cut into pieces

- 1 small lemon, thinly sliced and seeds removed

- 2 tablespoons chopped fresh basil, plus more for garnish

Directions

1. Sprinkle salt and pepper evenly over the chicken. Heat 1 tablespoon margarine in a huge nonstick skillet over medium intensity until foaming. Add the chicken; cook for about 3 minutes on each side, or

until browned and cooked through. Cover the chicken and place it on a plate to keep it warm.

2. Return the container to medium intensity. Add the excess 1 tablespoon spread and twirl to cover. Add garlic; cook, mixing continually, until fragrant, around 1 moment. Add stock and heat to the point of boiling over medium-high intensity. Add cream cheddar; cook, mixing continually, until dissolved and thickened, around 5 minutes. Mix in lemon cuts and basil. Return the chicken and any aggregated juices to the dish; stew over medium intensity until the sauce thickens and covers the chicken, around 4 minutes.

Nutrition Facts
(per serving)
236 Calories
12g Fat
2g Carbs
29g Protein

Squash And Red Lentil Curry

Cook Time: 15 mins
Additional Time: 25 mins
Total Time: 40 mins
Servings: 5
Yield: 5 servings

Ingredients

- 2 tablespoons canola oil

- 1 ½ cups diced onion

- 2 cloves garlic, minced

- 1 tablespoon minced fresh ginger

- 2 teaspoons curry powder or garam masala

- 1 20-ounce package cubed peeled butternut squash (see Tip)

- 1 cup red lentils

- 1 cup chopped fresh tomato or one 15-ounce can diced tomatoes, drained

- 1 ½ teaspoons salt

- 4 cups water

- 1 14-ounce can lite coconut milk

- 5 lime wedges

- Chopped fresh cilantro for garnish

Directions

1. Heat oil in a huge pot over medium-high intensity. Add onion, garlic, ginger and curry powder (or garam masala); cook, blending frequently, until the onion is beginning to mellow, 2 to 3 minutes. Salt, squash, lentils, and tomato cook, mixing, for 1 moment. Add water. Cover and heat to the point of boiling over high intensity. Lessen intensity to keep an energetic stew; Cover and cook for about 20 minutes, stirring occasionally, until the lentils are mostly broken down and the squash is tender.

2. Mix in coconut milk and stew until warmed through, around 1 moment. Present with lime wedges and cilantro, whenever wanted. Present with earthy colored rice or naan bread.

Tips:

Precut butternut squash is normally sold in a 20-ounce bundle of enormous 3D squares (5 cups of 1-to 2-inch pieces) or in a 16-ounce bundle of more modest diced squash (3 cups of 1/2-inch pieces). On the off chance that you can find the more modest 3D squares for this recipe, you'll have to purchase two 16-ounce bundles to have 5 complete cups of squash and lessen the simmering time by 5 to 10 minutes. Or on the other hand, you could prepare your own 3D shapes of squash from an entire, stripped and cultivated butternut at any point.

Nutrition Facts
(per serving)
326 Calories
12g Fat
47g Carbs
14g Protein

CHAPTER 6: VEGGIES AND SALAD SENSATION

Shrimp And Avocado Salad

Active Time:15 mins
Total Time:15 mins
Servings: 6

Ingredients

- 1 pound large peeled, deveined cooked shrimp, coarsely chopped

- 3 small ripe avocados, cubed

- ½ cup thinly sliced radishes

- ¼ cup thinly sliced scallions

- ¼ cup extra-virgin olive oil

- ¼ cup fresh lime juice

- 1 tablespoon grated fresh ginger

- 2 teaspoons granulated sugar

- ¾ teaspoon salt

- ¼ teaspoon crushed red pepper

- 12 cups mixed greens or chopped romaine lettuce

- Chopped fresh cilantro for garnish

Directions

Tenderly mix shrimp, avocados, radishes and scallions together in a medium bowl. Whisk oil, lime juice, ginger, sugar, salt and crushed red pepper in a little bowl. Pour the dressing over the shrimp combination; delicately mix to cover well. Partition greens (or lettuce) among 6 plates; Sprinkle evenly with the shrimp mixture and, if desired, cilantro for a garnish.

Nutrition Facts

(per serving)
367 Calories
25g Fat
17g Carbs
21g Protein

Taco Pasta Salad

Prep Time:15 mins
Additional Time:30 mins
Total Time:45 mins
Servings:8
Yield: 8 servings

Ingredients

- 12 ounces whole-wheat penne

- 2 cups shredded rotisserie chicken

- 1 pint grape tomatoes, halved

- 2 avocados, chopped

- 1 cup shredded sharp Cheddar cheese

- 1 cup thinly sliced red onion

- ¼ cup chopped fresh cilantro, plus more for garnish

- ⅓ cup salsa

- ¼ cup mayonnaise

- ¼ cup reduced-fat sour cream

- 2 tablespoons lime juice

- ½ teaspoon salt

- ½ teaspoon ground pepper

- ½ teaspoon ground cumin

- ¼ teaspoon chili powder

Directions

1. Cook pasta as per bundle headings. Flush with cold water; move to an enormous bowl. Mix in chicken, tomatoes, avocados, cheddar, onion and cilantro.

2. Whisk salsa, mayonnaise, sharp cream, lime juice, salt, pepper, cumin and bean stew powder in a little bowl. Add to the pasta blend and throw to cover. Refrigerate, covered, for 30 minutes or as long as 1 day (if holding for longer than 30 minutes, stand by to add avocados and cilantro until prepared to serve). Decorate with extra cilantro and serve.

Tips

To make ahead: Exclude avocados and cilantro and refrigerate for as long as 1 day. Mix in avocados and cilantro not long prior to serving.

Nutrition Facts

(per serving)
429 Calories
17g Fat
46g Carbs
25g Protein

Grilled Chicken Salad

Active Time:45 mins
Total Time:45 mins
Servings:6

Ingredients

- 1 small red onion

- 5 tablespoons red-wine vinegar, divided

- 2 medium cloves garlic, grated

- 1 teaspoon Dijon mustard

- 1 ½ teaspoons salt, divided

- ⅔ cup grapeseed oil, plus more for grill grates

- ½ teaspoon paprika

- 1 medium zucchini, sliced lengthwise into 1/2-inch-thick planks

- 1 small yellow bell pepper, cut into 2-inch-thick strips

- 2 large romaine lettuce hearts, halved lengthwise

- 3 (8 ounce) boneless, skinless chicken breasts

- 1 (5 ounce) package fresh baby spinach

- 2 small tomatoes, cut into 1-inch wedges

Directions

1. Preheat the barbecue to medium-high (400°F to 450°F). Divide the onion the long way through the root end. Cut 1 half into 1-inch wedges; put away. Meagerly cut the other half. Place the onion cuts in a little bowl; add 2 tablespoons vinegar; toss for a mix. Put away to pickle, blending incidentally, until prepared to utilize. Before serving, drain.

2. In a large bowl, whisk together the garlic, mustard, 1 teaspoon of salt, and the remaining 3 tablespoons of vinegar until the salt is dissolved. Gradually shower in oil, whisking continually, until the dressing is velvety. Put away 1/4 cup dressing. Mix paprika into the excess dressing in the bowl. Join zucchini cuts, ringer pepper strips, romaine parts and the held onion wedges on an enormous rimmed baking sheet. Sprinkle with half a cup of dressing; throw to cover well, trying to get dressing between the lettuce leaves. Place chicken in the enormous bowl with the excess dressing; throw to cover. Sprinkle with the excess 1/2 teaspoon salt.

3. Oil the barbecue grates by holding an oil-splashed paper towel with utensils. Barbecue the chicken and the vegetables, uncovered, for 1 moment. Keep barbecuing until the romaine is somewhat shriveled, around briefly more; move the romaine to the baking sheet. Keep barbecuing the chicken and vegetables, covered and turning at times, until the vegetables are delicately fresh with barbecue marks and a thermometer embedded into the thickest piece of chicken registers 165°F, around 6 minutes for the vegetables and 8 to 10 minutes for the

chicken. Return the barbecued chicken and vegetables to the baking sheet with the romaine; Before slicing, allow the chicken to rest for five minutes. Cut the vegetables and romaine into 1-inch-thick chunks.

4. Move the hacked romaine to an enormous bowl. Add spinach and the saved 1/4 cup dressing; throw well. Organize the combination on an enormous platter; top with cut chicken, zucchini, chime pepper, tomatoes and cured onions. Serve right away.

Nutrition Facts
(per serving)
416 Calories
26g Fat
16g Carbs
31g Protein

Strawberry Chicken Salad With Mint And Goat Cheese

Prep Time:40 mins
Total Time: 40 mins
Servings:4
Yield: 4 servings

Ingredients

- 1 pound chicken cutlets

- 6 tablespoons olive oil, divided

- ¾ teaspoon salt, divided

- ½ teaspoon ground pepper, divided

- 3 tablespoons white-wine vinegar

- 1 tablespoon minced shallot

- 1 ½ teaspoons honey

- 1 cup fresh mint leaves, divided, plus more for garnish

- 10 cups mixed salad greens (about 8 oz.)

- 2 ½ cups strawberries, sliced

- 4 ounces sugar snap peas, trimmed and thinly sliced

- 2 ounces goat cheese, crumbled (1/2 cup)

- ¼ cup sliced almonds, toasted

Directions

1. Preheat the barbecue to medium-high. (No barbecue? See Tip.) Brush chicken with 1 Tbsp. sprinkle with 1/4 teaspoon oil. each salt and pepper. Barbecue, turning once, until cooked through, 2 to 3 minutes for each side. At the point when sufficiently cool to deal with, cut the chicken.

2. In the meantime, whisk vinegar, shallot, honey, and the excess 5 Tbsp. oil, 1/2 tsp. salt, and 1/4 tsp. pepper in a huge bowl. Chop 1/4 cup of mint finely; add to the dressing in the bowl, speeding to join. Hold 2 Tbsp. of the covering

3. Tear or coarsely hack the leftover 3/4 cup mint leaves; add to the bowl alongside blended greens. Throw delicately to join. Split the plate of mixed greens between 4 super bowls. Consolidate the chicken and the saved 2 Tbsp. dressing in the enormous bowl; toss to combine. Partition the chicken, strawberries, snap peas, goat cheddar, and almonds among the 4 super bowls. Embellish with more mint, whenever wanted.

TIps:

Preheat the grill excessively high. Plan chicken as coordinated in Sync 1 and cook on a huge baking sheet 3 to 4 crawls from the intensity source, flipping once, until it arrives at an inner temperature of 165 degrees F, 4 to 6 minutes for every side.

Nutrition Facts
(per serving)
442 Calories
29g Fat
17g Carbs
30g Protein

Chili-Rubbed Flank Steak Salad

Prep Time: 55 mins
Additional Time: 1 hr 50 mins
Total Time: 2 hrs 45 mins
Servings: 4
Yield: 4 servings

Ingredients
Steak And Rub

- 1 pound flank steak, trimmed

- 2 tablespoons avocado oil or canola oil

- 1 clove garlic, minced

- 1 tablespoon chili powder

- 1 teaspoon unsweetened cocoa powder

- 1 teaspoon ground cumin

- ½ teaspoon ground cinnamon

- ½ teaspoon ground pepper

- ¼ teaspoon salt

Dressing

- ¼ cup loosely packed fresh cilantro, finely chopped

- ¼ cup low-fat plain Greek yogurt

- 2 tablespoons mayonnaise

- 1 teaspoon lime zest

- 2 tablespoons lime juice

- 1 clove garlic, minced

- 1 teaspoon honey

- ⅛ teaspoon salt

Salad

- 6 cups chopped romaine lettuce

- 1 cup frozen corn kernels, thawed

- 1 (15 ounce) can low-sodium black beans, rinsed

- 1 large orange or yellow bell pepper, thinly sliced

- ½ medium red onion, thinly sliced

- ¼ cup crumbled feta cheese

- ¼ cup chopped fresh cilantro

- 2 tablespoons pepitas

Directions

1. To plan steak and rub: In a large glass dish, place the steak. Join oil, garlic, stew powder, cocoa, cumin, cinnamon, pepper, and 1/4 tsp. salt in a little bowl. Apply the mixture to the steak on both sides. Cover and refrigerate for 1 1/2 to 2 hours.

2. In the interim, plan dressing: Whisk cilantro, yogurt, mayonnaise, lime zing, lime juice, garlic, honey, and salt in a different bowl.

3. To cook steak: Preheat barbecue to medium-high. Clean and oil the meshes (see Tip). Barbecue the steak to want doneness, 4 to 5 minutes for every side for seared to perfection (130-135 degrees F on a moment read thermometer). Before slicing, transfer to a clean cutting board and allow to rest for four to five minutes.

4. To plan salad: Join lettuce, corn, beans, ringer pepper, and onion in an enormous bowl. Add the dressing and throw to cover.

5. Cut the steak daintily across the grain. Split the serving of mixed greens between 4 plates, top with the steak, and sprinkle with feta, cilantro, and pepitas, if utilizing.

Tips

- To make ahead: Refrigerate dressing (Stage 2) for as long as 2 days.

- To oil a hot barbecue grind, splash a paper towel with vegetable oil, hold it with utensils and rub it over the mesh. (Try not to utilize cooking splash on a hot barbecue.)

Nutrition Facts
(per serving)
467 Calories
22g Fat
32g Carbs
36g Protein

CHAPTER 7: **COOKIE AND DESSERT RECIPES**

Cranberry-Coconut Oatmeal Cookies

Active Time:15 mins
Total Time:30 mins
Servings:12

Ingredients

- 1 large egg

- ½ cup granulated sugar

- ⅔ cup rolled oats

- 3 ½ tablespoons unsweetened coconut flakes, crushed

- 2 tablespoons finely chopped dried cranberries

- 2 teaspoons melted butter

- ¼ teaspoon salt

- ¼ teaspoon vanilla extract

- ⅛ teaspoon lemon extract

Directions

1. Preheat the broiler to 325°F. Cover a baking sheet with a cooking shower.

2. Beat egg in a medium bowl. Steadily add sugar, mixing to join. Add oats, coconut, cranberries, spread, salt, vanilla and lemon separate; mix until completely consolidated. Drop the mixture by the teaspoonful onto the

   pre-arranged baking sheet, around 1 1/2 inches separated. Spread every mixture hill into a round shape utilizing a fork plunged in chilly water.

3. Prepare until gently caramelized, 10 to 15 minutes. After three minutes on the baking sheet, transfer to a wire rack to cool completely.

Tips

Individuals with celiac infection or gluten responsiveness ought to utilize oats that are named "sans gluten," as oats are many times cross-debased with wheat and grain.

Nutrition Facts

(per serving)
74 Calories
2g Fat
13g Carbs
1g Protein

<u>**Vegan Chocolate Chip Cookies**</u>

Prep Time: 20 mins
Additional Time: 1 hr 5 mins
Total Time: 1 hr 25 mins
Servings:15
Yield: 30 cookies

Ingredients

- 1 cup white whole-wheat flour

- 1 cup all-purpose flour

- 1 ½ teaspoons baking powder

- ¼ teaspoon baking soda

- ½ teaspoon salt

- ⅔ cup packed light brown sugar

- ½ cup coconut oil, melted

- ½ cup warm water

- ⅓ cup unsalted smooth almond butter

- 2 teaspoons vanilla extract

- ⅔ cup vegan chocolate chips, preferably bittersweet

Directions

1. Whisk white entire wheat flour, regular flour, baking powder, baking pop and salt in a medium bowl. Whisk sugar, coconut oil, water, almond spread and vanilla in a huge bowl. Add the flour blend to the sugar combination and mix until recently joined. Overlay in chocolate chips. Cover the bowl and let it stand at room temperature for something like 30 minutes.

2. Prepare a baking sheet with parchment paper and preheat the oven to 350 degrees Fahrenheit. Utilizing around 1 loading tablespoon for every treat, drop hills of mixture, something like 1 inch separated, on the pre-arranged baking sheet. Level the hills to make 2 far reaching treats. Prepare until delicately sautéed, 10 to 14 minutes. After cooling for two minutes on the baking sheet, transfer the cookies to a rack to cool completely. Rehash with the excess mixture.

Nutrition Facts
(per serving)
231 Calories
13g Fat
28g Carbs
3g Protein

<u>Banana Chocolate Chip Mini Muffins</u>

Prep Time:20 mins
Additional Time:30 mins
Total Time:50 mins
Servings:24
Yield: 24 muffins

Ingredients

- 1 ½ cups rolled oats (see Tip)

- 1 teaspoon baking powder

- ¼ teaspoon baking soda

- ¼ teaspoon salt

- 2 large eggs

- 1 cup mashed ripe banana (about 2 medium-large)

- ⅓ cup packed brown sugar

- 3 tablespoons canola oil

- 1 teaspoon vanilla extract

- ½ cup mini chocolate chips

Directions

1. Preheat the oven to 350 degrees F. Cover a 24-cup smaller than expected biscuit tin with cooking splash.

2. Beat oats in a blender until finely ground. Add baking powder, baking pop and salt; Blend by pulsing once or twice. Combine the brown sugar, eggs, banana, oil, and vanilla; puree until smooth. Mix in chocolate chips. Fill the pre-arranged biscuit cups.

3. Prepare until a toothpick embedded in the middle tells the truth, 15 to 17 minutes. Cool in the container on a wire rack for 5 minutes, then, at that point, end up cooling totally..

Nutrition Facts
(per serving)
78 Calories
4g Fat
11g Carbs
1g Protein

Lemon-Blueberry Bars

Active Time:15 mins
Total Time:2 hrs 40 mins
Servings:9

Ingredients

- 1 ¼ cups graham cracker crumbs

- 4 tablespoons salted butter, melted

- 1 tablespoon granulated sugar

- Zest of 1 lemon, divided

- 1 (14 ounce) can sweetened condensed milk

- ½ cup lemon juice

- 1 large egg

- 1 cup fresh blueberries

Directions

1. Preheat the oven to 350°F. Cover a 8-inch-square baking dish with a cooking shower.

2. Mix graham wafer pieces, spread, sugar and a portion of the lemon zing together in a medium bowl. Press the blend solidly and equally into the pre-arranged container. Prepare until gently sautéed around

the edges, around 10 minutes. Set aside to cool for at least 10 minutes on a wire rack in the pan.

3. In the meantime, completely whisk dense milk, lemon juice, egg and the leftover lemon zing together in a medium bowl. Mix in blueberries. Over the baked crust, distribute the filling evenly. Heat until set, 16 to 18 minutes. Let cool at room temperature for 60 minutes. Cover and refrigerate for something like 1 hour more.

Nutrition Facts
(per serving)
273 Calories
11g Fat
40g Carbs
5g Protein

Apple-Pie Baked Oats

Active Time: 25 mins
Total Time:1 hr
Servings:6

Ingredients

- 2 tablespoons unsalted butter

- 2 large firm sweet apples, such as Honeycrisp, thinly sliced

- 1 teaspoon ground cinnamon

- ¼ cup brown sugar

- 2 cups whole milk

- 2 large eggs

- 3 cups rolled oats

- 3 tablespoons vanilla protein powder, such as BioSteel

- 2 tablespoons chia seeds

- 1 teaspoon baking powder

- Plain Greek yogurt & pure maple syrup for serving

Directions

1. Preheat the oven to 375°F. Spray cooking spray into a baking dish that is 9 by 13 inches. Liquefy margarine in a 10-inch skillet over medium-low intensity. Cook, stirring, for one to two minutes after adding the sliced apples, until well coated. Add cinnamon; cook, blending, until the cinnamon is toasted and fragrant, 1 to 2 minutes. Add earthy colored sugar; cook, stirring frequently, for 3 to 5 minutes or until the apples are soft.

2. Whisk milk and eggs in an enormous bowl. Mix in oats, protein powder, chia seeds and baking powder. Add the apple combination and mix to join.

3. Move the hitter to the pre-arranged baking dish, spreading it uniformly. Heat until brilliant brown on the edges, 30 to 35 minutes. Put the container on a wire rack to cool somewhat, around 10 minutes, prior to cutting into 6 cuts. Top each present with a spot of yogurt or potentially a sprinkle of maple syrup, whenever wanted.

Nutrition Facts

(per serving)

361 Calories

12g Fat

53g Carbs

12g Protein

<u>**Sugar Free Strawberry Cream**</u>

Prep Time: 15 mins
Additional Time:12 hrs 15 mins
Total Time: 12 hrs 30 mins
Servings:4
Yield: 4 cups

Ingredients

- 1 pound fresh strawberries

- 2 medium bananas

- 1 tablespoon fresh lemon juice

- ¼ cup ice-cold water, as needed

Directions

1. Strawberries can be hulled and chopped coarsely. Strip and coarsely cleave bananas. Spread the strawberries and bananas on independent sides of one baking sheet or on two sheets. Freeze until strong, somewhere around 12 hours.

2. Allow the strawberries to defrost at room temperature for 15 minutes. Move to a food processor; roughly 10 pulses until finely chopped Include the lemon juice and frozen bananas; process until smooth, 1 to 1 1/2 minutes, amounting to 1/4 cup cold water if necessary to accomplish wanted consistency, halting to scratch disadvantages of bowl on a case by case basis. Serve right away or, for a firmer surface, move to a cooler safe holder and freeze for as long as 30 minutes..

Nutrition Facts
(per serving)
191 Calories
1g Fat
23g Carbs
1g Protein

Sugar Free Pineapple Cream

Prep Time:5 mins
Total Time:5 mins
Servings:6
Yield:3 cups

Ingredients

- 1 16-ounce package frozen pineapple chunks

- 1 cup frozen mango chunks or 1 large mango, peeled, seeded and chopped

- 1 tablespoon lemon juice or lime juice

Directions

- In a food processor, blend pineapple, mango, and lemon (or lime) juice until smooth and creamy. (In the case of utilizing frozen mango, you might need to amount to 1/4 cup water.) For the best surface, serve right away.

Nutrition Facts

(per serving)
55 Calories
0g Fat
14g Carbs
1g Protein

Diabetes-Friendly Carrot Cake

Active Time:
45 mins
Additional Time:
25 mins
Total Time:
1 hr 10 mins
Servings:
14
Yield:
14 servings

Ingredients
Carrot Cake

- 1 ½ cups all-purpose flour

- ⅔ cup flax-seed meal

- 2 teaspoons baking powder

- 1 teaspoon pumpkin pie spice

- ½ teaspoon baking soda

- ¼ teaspoon salt

- 3 cups finely shredded carrot (about 6 medium carrots) (see Tip)

- 1 cup refrigerated or frozen egg product, thawed, or 4 eggs, lightly beaten

- ½ cup granulated sugar (see Tip)

- ½ cup packed brown sugar (see Tip)

- ½ cup canola oil

- 1 Coarsely shredded carrot

Fluffy Cream Cheese Frosting

- 2 ounces softened reduced-fat cream cheese (Neufchâtel)

- ½ teaspoon vanilla

- ¼ cup powdered sugar

- 1 ½ cups frozen light-whipped dessert topping

Directions

1. Set the oven's temperature to 350 degrees. Pat two 8x1-1/2- or 9x1-1/2-inch round cake pans dry with grease and dust with flour. Use parchment paper or waxed paper to line the bottoms. Grease and dust the sides of the pans that have been lined with parchment or wax paper. Put aside.

2. Mix together flour, flax seed meal, baking powder, pumpkin pie spice, baking soda, and salt in a large mixing dish. Put aside. Add the eggs, brown sugar, granulated sugar, oil, and finely shredded carrots to

another large mixing basin. Add the egg mixture to the flour mixture right away. Mix well until well combined. Distribute the batter equally among the pans that have been prepared.

3. For 8-inch pans, bake for 25–30 minutes; for 9-inch pans, bake for 20–25 minutes, or until a toothpick inserted in the center comes out clean. Allow cakes in pans to cool for ten minutes on wire racks. Turn cakes out onto wire stands. Let cool fully.

4. Reduced-fat cream cheese (Neufchâtel) should be smoothed out in a medium bowl using an electric mixer set to medium to high speed. Mix in the vanilla. Add powdered sugar gradually while beating until smooth. Defrost 1-1/2 cups of frozen light whipped topping for dessert. To lighten, fold in approximately 1/2 cup of the topping into the cream cheese mixture. Incorporate the leftover whipped topping.

5. Arrange one cake layer, cooled, onto a dish for serving. Cover with half of the frosting made of fluffy cream cheese. Spread the leftover frosting over the second cake layer that has been placed atop the frosting. Sprinkle some roughly shredded carrot on top, if you'd like.

Tips:

- To keep the carrots from baking all the way to the bottom of the pan, make sure you shred them thinly.

- When substituting sugar, use Splenda(R) Sugar Blend for Baking rather than granulated sugar. Instead of using brown sugar, use Splenda(R) Brown Sugar Blend for Baking. Use product amount equal to 1/2 cup granulated and brown sugar, following package guidelines. Per serving nutrition analysis: same as below, excluding 231 calories, 25 grams of carbohydrates, and 186 milligrams of salt.

Values per day: 3% calcium. 1 1/2 additional carbs are exchanged. Options for carbohydrates: 1 ½.

Nutrition Facts
(per serving)
254 Calories
12g Fat
34g Carbs
5g Protein

Frozen Strawberry-Chocolate Yogurt Bark

Active Time: 10 mins
Additional Time:3 hrs
Total Time: 3 hrs 10 mins
Servings:32
Yield: 32 pieces

Ingredients

- 3 cups whole-milk plain Greek yogurt

- ¼ cup pure maple syrup or honey

- 1 teaspoon vanilla extract

- 1 ½ cups sliced strawberries

- ¼ cup mini chocolate chips

Directions

1. Line a huge rimmed baking sheet with material paper.

2. In a medium bowl, combine yogurt, vanilla, and maple syrup (or honey). Spread into a 10-by-15-inch rectangle on the baking sheet that has been prepared. Sprinkle chocolate chips and scatter the strawberries over the top.

3. Freeze until extremely firm, something like 3 hours. Cut or split into 32 pieces to serve.

Nutrition Facts
(per serving)
34 Calories
1g Fat
4g Carbs
2g Protein

<u>**Whipped Frozen Lemonade**</u>

Active Time: 10 mins
Additional Time:1 hr
Total Time: 1 hr 10 mins
Servings:4
Yield: 4 cocktails

Ingredients

- Lemon Simple Syrup

- ½ cup granulated sugar

- ½ cup water

- Zest of 1 lemon

- Lemonade

- ½ cup freshly squeezed lemon juice (from 2 lemons)

- 1 cup full-fat coconut milk

- 2 ½ cups ice cubes

Directions

1. Making simple syrup: Carry sugar and water to a stew in a little pot over medium intensity, mixing every so often until the sugar disintegrates. Mix in lemon zing and eliminate from heat. Cover and let steep for 60 minutes, then, at that point, strain the syrup through a

fine-network sifter; dispose of the zing. (There will be extra syrup; refrigerate for as long as several weeks.)

2. To get ready whipped lemonade: Add 1/2 cup straightforward syrup, lemon juice, coconut milk and ice to a blender. Mix until the ice is squashed and the blend is slushy. Split between 4 8-ounce glasses and serve right away.

Nutrition Facts
(per serving)
167 Calories
12g Fat
16g Carbs
1g Protein

CHAPTER 8: **SEAFOOD FEAST**

Crispy Baked Catfish

Active Time:10 mins
Total Time:25 mins
Servings:4

Ingredients

- Cooking spray

- ½ cup fine plain yellow cornmeal

- ¼ cup all-purpose flour

- 1 tablespoon salt free Cajun seasoning

- 1 large egg

- 4 (5 ounce) catfish filets

- ½ teaspoon salt

- Tartar sauce and lemon wedges (optional)

Directions

1. Set the oven temperature to 450°F. Line an enormous rimmed baking sheet with foil and top with a wire rack. Cover the rack with a cooking splash.

2. Mix cornmeal, flour and Cajun-Creole flavoring mix together in an enormous shallow dish. Whisk egg in a different shallow dish.

3. Wipe filets off with a paper towel and sprinkle equally with salt. Working with 1 filet at a time, dip in the egg to cover, allowing the overabundant egg to dribble once more into the dish. Then dig in the cornmeal combination, going to cover the two sides. Move to the pre-arranged rack on the baking sheet. Rehash with the leftover filets. Cover the highest points of the filets with cooking splash.

4. Bread shop until fresh and brilliant, 15 to 20 minutes, turning the filets over and covering with cooking splash part of the way through. Whenever wanted, present with tartar sauce and lemon wedges.

Nutrition Facts
(per serving)
232 Calories
7g Fat
11g Carbs
30g Protein

Almond And Lemon-Crusted Fish With Spinach

Cook Time:25 mins
Total Time:25 mins
Servings:4
Yield:4 servings

Ingredients
- Zest and juice of 1 lemon, divided

- ½ cup sliced almonds, coarsely chopped

- 1 tablespoon finely chopped fresh dill or 1 teaspoon dried

- 1 tablespoon plus 2 teaspoons extra-virgin olive oil, divided

- 1 teaspoon kosher salt, divided

- Freshly ground pepper to taste

- 1 1/4 pounds cod (see Tip) or halibut, cut into 4 portions

- 4 teaspoons Dijon mustard

- 2 cloves garlic, slivered

- 1 pound baby spinach

- Lemon wedges for garnish

Directions

1. Preheat the oven to 400 degrees F. Cover a rimmed baking sheet with cooking splash.

2. In a small bowl, combine the almonds, dill, lemon zest, 1 tablespoon oil, and 1/2 teaspoon each of salt and pepper. Put fish on the pre-arranged baking sheet and spread each part with 1 teaspoon mustard. Split the almond combination between the segments, compressing it onto the mustard.

3. Depending on the thickness, bake the fish for 7 to 9 minutes or until opaque in the middle.

4. In the meantime, heat the leftover 2 teaspoons of oil in a Dutch broiler over medium intensity. Add garlic and cook, mixing, until fragrant yet not brown, around 30 seconds. Add spinach, the juice from the lemon, and the remaining 1/2 teaspoon of salt; pepper the dish. Cook, blending frequently, until the spinach is recently withered, 2 to 4 minutes. Cover to keep warm. If desired, serve the fish with lemon wedges and spinach.

Nutrition Facts

(per serving)
244 Calories
12g Fat
8g Carbs
27g Protein

Salmon Noodle Casserole

Active Time: 1 hr
Total Time: 2 hrs
Servings: 6

Ingredients

- 8 ounces whole-wheat egg noodles

- 1 cup sliced fresh asparagus

- 2 tablespoons extra-virgin olive oil plus 1 teaspoon, divided

- 1 medium leek, halved lengthwise and thinly sliced crosswise

- 2 teaspoons minced garlic

- ¼ cup all-purpose flour

- 3 ½ cups whole milk

- 1 tablespoon Dijon mustard

- ½ teaspoon salt

- ½ teaspoon ground pepper

- ¼ teaspoon cayenne pepper

- 2 (6 ounce) cans no-salt-added boneless, skinless pink salmon, drained and flaked

- 1 cup frozen peas, thawed

- ½ cup whole-wheat panko breadcrumbs

- ½ cup shredded white Cheddar cheese

- 1 tablespoon finely chopped fresh flat-leaf parsley

Directions

1. Preheat the stove to 375°F. Heat a huge pot of water to the point of boiling over high intensity. Noodles, please; cook for about 5 minutes, stirring occasionally, until the noodles are slightly softened but still somewhat firm. Add asparagus; cook, blending frequently, until the asparagus is dazzling green and delicate fresh and the noodles are completely cooked, around 2 minutes. Channel and put away.

2. Clean the pot off. Add 2 tablespoons of oil and intensity over medium-high intensity. Include leek cook, blending incidentally, until relaxed and clear, around 5 minutes. Add garlic; cook, blending frequently, until fragrant, around 1 moment. Sprinkle flour over it. Lessen intensity to medium and cook, blending continually, for 2 minutes. Steadily add milk, racing until smooth. Bring to a delicate bubble over medium-high intensity, whisking frequently. Turn down the heat to medium-low; delicately stew, whisking frequently, until thickened, around 5 minutes. Eliminate from heat. Add mustard, cayenne, salt, and pepper; mix well with a whisk. Add the noodle-asparagus blend, salmon and peas; overlap until the noodles

are completely covered. Spread the combination uniformly in a 2-quart baking dish.

3. Join panko, cheddar, parsley and the leftover 1 teaspoon oil in a medium bowl; mix until very much blended. Sprinkle uniformly over the meal. In about 15 minutes, bake until the topping is golden brown and the cheese has melted. Let represent 5 minutes prior to serving.

Nutrition Facts
(per serving)
441 Calories
15g Fat
47g Carbs
25g Protein

<u>**Shrimp Tacos**</u>

Prep Time: 30 mins
Total Time: 30 mins
Servings:4
Yield: 8 cups

Ingredients

- 2 cups diced tomatoes

- 1 teaspoon lime zest (reserve before juicing limes)

- 5 tablespoons lime juice, divided

- ¼ cup chopped fresh cilantro

- ¼ cup diced red onion

- 2 tablespoons minced jalapeño pepper

- ⅛ teaspoon salt

- 2 tablespoons tahini

- ½ teaspoon honey

- 1 clove garlic, minced

- 2 tablespoons olive oil

- 1 tablespoon ground cumin

- 2 teaspoons ground coriander

- ¼ teaspoon ground pepper

- 1 pound large raw shrimp (21-25 count; see Tip), peeled and deveined

- 8 (6 inch) flour tortillas, warmed

- 1 cup thinly sliced radishes

Directions

1. Preheat the oven. Join tomatoes, 2 Tbsp. lime juice, cilantro, onion, jalapeño, and salt in a medium bowl; throw to consolidate.

2. Whisk lime zing, the excess 3 Tbsp. lime juice, tahini, honey, and garlic in a little bowl.

3. Consolidate oil, cumin, coriander, and pepper in an enormous bowl. Add shrimp and throw to cover. Spread the shrimp on an enormous rimmed baking sheet. Sear, flipping once, until the shrimp are pink and just cooked through, 4 to 6 minutes.

4. To collect: Each tortilla should have 2 to 3 shrimp on it. Add about 3 Tbsp to each. 2 teaspoons salsa tahini sauce, and 2 Tbsp. radishes.

Nutrition Facts
(per serving)
398 Calories
16g Fat
34g Carbs
29g Protein

Garlic Shrimp And Rice

Active Time: 25 mins
Total Time: 35 mins
Servings:4

Ingredients
- 3 small scallions

- 5 medium cloves garlic, divided

- 2 tablespoons extra-virgin olive oil

- 2 small bell peppers, chopped

- 2 teaspoons grated lemon zest

- ¼ teaspoon crushed red pepper

- 1 cup long-grain white rice

- 2 cups water

- ½ teaspoon salt

- 12 ounces medium peeled, deveined raw shrimp

- 2 tablespoons butter

- 2 teaspoons lemon juice

- Lemon wedges, for serving

Directions

1. Cut white and light green pieces of scallions; put away. Daintily cut dull green scallion parts; put away. Meagerly cut 4 garlic cloves; place aside. Grind the leftover garlic clove utilizing a Microplane grater; put away.

2. Heat oil in a huge, profound nonstick skillet with a tight-fitting top over medium-high intensity. Add the white and light green scallion cuts, ringer peppers, lemon zing, crushed red pepper and the cut garlic. Cook, mixing sometimes, until the peppers somewhat relax, 5 to 6 minutes. Add rice; cook, mixing continually, for 1 moment. Mix in water and salt; carry the blend to a stew over medium-high intensity. Cover and diminish intensity to low. Cook, undisturbed, until the rice is delicate, around 20 minutes, orchestrating shrimp on top of the blend (don't mix in) during the last 5 minutes of cook time. Eliminate from heat; let stand, covered, until the shrimp are cooked through, around 5 minutes.

3. In a small microwave-safe bowl, combine the grated garlic, lemon juice, and butter. Microwave on High until the spread is liquefied, around 25 seconds. Mix the blend and shower over the shrimp. Sprinkle with the held dim green scallion cuts. Cushion the rice (don't mix in the shrimp) utilizing a fork. Present with lemon wedges, whenever wanted.

Nutrition Facts
(per serving)
383 Calories
14g Fat
47g Carbs
17g Protein

Lobster Ravioli

Prep Time:25 mins
Total Time:25 mins
Servings:2
Yield:2 servings

Ingredients

- 1 ½ teaspoons all-purpose flour

- ½ cup whole milk, divided

- ¼ cup frozen peas, thawed

- 1 teaspoon chopped fresh tarragon

- ¼ teaspoon lemon zest

- ¾ teaspoon lemon juice

- ⅛ teaspoon kosher salt

- ⅛ teaspoon ground pepper

- 1 ½ tablespoons finely minced fresh chives, divided

- 1 (9 ounce) package refrigerated lobster ravioli (such as Trader Joe's)

- 3 ounces cooked lobster meat (Optional)

Directions

1. Whisk flour and 1/4 cup milk in a little bowl until smooth. In a small saucepan, bring the remaining 1/4 cup of milk just to a boil over medium heat. Race in the flour blend; stew, whisking continually, until somewhat thickened, around 1 moment. Take off the heat. Mix in peas, tarragon, lemon zing, lemon juice, salt, pepper and 1 tablespoon chives. Keep warm, covered, until you're ready to serve.

2. In the meantime, get ready ravioli as per bundle headings; drain. Partition the ravioli equally among 2 shallow dishes; top with the sauce, lobster (if utilizing) and the leftover 1/2 tablespoon chives.

Nutrition Facts
(per serving)
348 Calories
10g Fat
48g Carbs
16g Protein

Salmon Potato Cakes

Cook Time:30 mins
Total Time:30 mins
Servings:2
Yield:2 servings, cakes each

Ingredients

- 1 teaspoon extra-virgin olive oil

- 1 ½ cups frozen hash brown potatoes, thawed

- 1 large egg white

- 1 tablespoon low-fat mayonnaise

- 2 teaspoons drained capers, coarsely chopped

- 1 scallion, trimmed and thinly sliced

- 1/8 teaspoon salt

- Freshly ground pepper, to taste

- 1 7-ounce can wild salmon, (see Ingredient Note), drained, picked over and flaked

Directions

1. Preheat the oven to 450 degrees F. To some extent squash potatoes in a bowl with a fork until they start to keep intact. Add salmon, egg

white, mayonnaise, escapades, scallion, salt and pepper. Shape the blend into 4 cakes, each around 1/2 inch thick.

2. Heat oil in an ovenproof nonstick skillet over medium intensity. Cook the salmon cakes for 4 to 5 minutes, or until they are browned on the bottom. Cautiously turn the cakes over with a spatula and move the dish to the stove. Prepare until warmed through and brilliant brown on the subsequent side, 5 to 7 minutes.

Nutrition Facts
(per serving)
323 Calories
13g Fat
31g Carbs
24g Protein

Air-Fryer Fish Cakes

Cook Time:10 mins
Active Time:10 mins
Total Time:20 mins
Servings:2
Yield:4 cakes

Ingredients

- Cooking spray

- 10 ounces finely chopped white fish (such as grouper, catfish or cod)

- ⅔ cup whole-wheat panko breadcrumbs

- 3 tablespoons finely chopped fresh cilantro

- 2 tablespoons Thai sweet chili sauce

- 2 tablespoons canola mayonnaise

- 1 large egg

- ⅛ teaspoon salt

- ¼ teaspoon ground pepper

- 2 lime wedges

Directions

1. Cover the crate of an air fryer with a cooking splash.

2. Consolidate fish, panko, cilantro, bean stew sauce, mayonnaise, egg, salt and pepper in a medium bowl; mix until very much consolidated. Shape the blend into four 3-inch-width cakes.

3. Cover the cakes with a cooking shower; place in the pre-arranged bushel. In 9 to 10 minutes, cook the cakes at 400 degrees F until they are browned and have an internal temperature of 140 degrees F. Present with lime wedges.

Nutrition Facts
(per serving)
399 Calories
16g Fat
28g Carbs
35g Protein

Grilled Salmon With Kale Saute

Prep Time: 25 mins
Additional Time: 20 mins
Total Time:45 mins
Servings:2
Yield:2 servings

Ingredients

- 2 (5 ounce) fresh or frozen skinless salmon filets, about 1 inch thick

- ½ teaspoon dried thyme, crushed

- ¼ teaspoon garlic powder

- ⅛ teaspoon salt

- ⅛ teaspoon cayenne pepper

- 1 tablespoon finely chopped shallot

- 1 small clove garlic, minced

- ½ teaspoon olive oil

- 6 ounces fresh kale, torn (discard stems)

- ½ teaspoon finely shredded lemon peel

- Dash salt

- Lemon wedges

Directions

1. Defrost fish, whenever frozen. Flush fish; wipe off with paper towels. Place aside. Combine the cayenne pepper, 1/8 teaspoon of salt, and thyme in a small bowl. Sprinkle the highest points of the filets equally with preparing the blend.

2. For a charcoal barbecue, put fish on the lubed barbecue rack straight over medium coals. Before placing the fish, cover the grill grate with foil if desired. Barbecue, uncovered, for 8 to 12 minutes or until fish starts to peel when tried with a fork, turning fish once partially through barbecuing. (Preheat the grill for a gas grill. Lessen intensity to medium. Put fish on a lubed barbecue rack over heat. Grill as directed with a cover.) Cover fish to keep warm.

3. Cook the shallot and garlic for 2 to 4 minutes, or until tender, in hot oil in a Dutch oven over medium heat. Add kale and lemon strips. Cover and cook for 2 minutes. Uncover and cook for 6 to 8 minutes more or just until kale starts to shrink, turning with long-dealt with utensils to cook. Sprinkle with the scramble salt. Serve salmon with kale and lemon wedges.

Nutrition Facts
(per serving)
357 Calories
21g Fat
11g Carbs
32g Protein

CHAPTER 9: **SAVORY SOUP AND STEW RECIPES**

Cabbage Soup

Prep Time:20 mins
Additional Time:40 mins
Total Time:1 hr
Servings:8
Yield:8 servings

Ingredients
- 2 tablespoons canola oil

- 1 ½ pounds lean ground beef

- 4 cups chopped green cabbage

- 2 cups chopped yellow onion

- 1 ¼ cups chopped carrots

- 1 cup chopped celery

- 2 tablespoons light brown sugar

- 1 tablespoon smoked paprika

- 1 teaspoon salt

- ½ teaspoon ground pepper

- ¼ teaspoon cayenne pepper

- 1 (15 ounce) can no-salt-added tomato sauce

- 4 cups unsalted chicken broth

- ¼ cup medium-grain brown rice

- 2 tablespoons chopped fresh flat-leaf parsley (optional)

Directions

1. Heat oil in an enormous weighty pot over medium-high intensity. Add beef ground up; cook, blending frequently, until the meat is cooked through and beginning to brown marginally, 6 to 7 minutes. Add cabbage, onion, carrots and celery; cook, mixing frequently, until the onion is clear, around 5 minutes.

2. Add earthy colored sugar, paprika, salt, pepper and cayenne to the meat blend; cook over medium-high intensity, blending continually, until the flavors are toasted, around 1 moment. Mix in pureed tomatoes and stock, scratching the lower part of the pot with a wooden spoon to deliver any seared pieces. Heat the soup to the point of boiling over medium-high intensity. Mix in rice. Turn heat down to low; cover and cook until the rice is delicate, 30 to 35 minutes. Whenever wanted, sprinkle with parsley prior to serving.

Nutrition Facts
(per serving)
300 Calories

17g Fat
18g Carbs
20g Protein

<u>**Chicken Soup**</u>

Prep Time:30 mins
Additional Time:15 mins
Total Time:45 mins
Servings:6
Yield: 9 cups

Ingredients
- 1 tablespoon canola oil

- 1 cup chopped onion

- 3 cloves garlic, minced

- 5 cups low-sodium chicken broth

- 1 (15 ounce) can diced tomatoes

- 1 (4 ounce) can diced green chiles

- 6 corn tortillas, chopped
- 2 teaspoons chili powder

- 1 teaspoon ground cumin

- 2 cups shredded cooked chicken breast

- 4 ounces reduced-fat cream cheese, softened

- ¾ cup shredded white Cheddar cheese

- 1 ½ teaspoons cornstarch

- Fresh cilantro, sour cream and/or guacamole for garnish

Directions

1. Heat oil in a huge pot over medium intensity. Add onion and cook, mixing every so often, until relaxed, around 3 minutes. Stir in the garlic and cook for one minute. Add stock, tomatoes, chiles, tortillas, bean stew powder and cumin. Heat to the point of boiling, mixing infrequently. Diminish intensity to a stew. Cover and cook for 20 minutes.

2. Add chicken and cream cheddar, blending until the cream cheddar is softened. Take off the heat. In a little bowl, join the destroyed cheddar and cornstarch. Gradually add the mixture to the soup and stir until melted. Return the pot to medium intensity and cook until hot, 1 to 2 minutes. Serve the soup with cilantro, acrid cream as well as guacamole, whenever wanted.

Nutrition Facts
(per serving)
329 Calories
15g Fat
23g Carbs
26g Protein

Vegetarian Lasagna Soup

Active Time:20 mins
Total Time:20 mins
Servings:4

Ingredients

- 2 tablespoons extra-virgin olive oil

- 3 ½ cups sliced cremini mushrooms

- 2 cups zucchini, cut into 1/3-inch-thick half-moons

- 1 tablespoon garlic paste

- 3 cups water

- 1 (24 ounce) jar low-sodium marinara sauce

- ¼ teaspoon salt

- 4 ounces lasagna noodles (about 4 to 5 noodles), preferably whole-wheat, broken into 1-inch pieces

- 3 cups baby spinach

- ½ cup whole-milk ricotta cheese

- ¼ cup shredded low-moisture whole-milk mozzarella-and-provolone blend

- 1 tablespoon grated Parmesan cheese (see Tip)

Directions

1. In a large pot, heat the oil to medium-high heat. Mix in mushrooms and zucchini; cook, blending frequently, until the vegetables are marginally mellowed, 3 to 5 minutes. Include the garlic paste; cook, blending continually, until fragrant, around 1 moment. Add water, marinara and salt; heat to the point of boiling over medium-high intensity. Add noodles and mix to separate, around 30 seconds. Cook, blending periodically, until the noodles are simply cooked through yet not totally delicate, 8 to 10 minutes. Add spinach; cook, blending incidentally, until recently withered, around 1 moment.

2. In the meantime, join ricotta, destroyed cheddar and Parmesan in a little bowl.

3. Split the soup between 4 dishes. Top each present with a bit of the ricotta combination.

Tips:

- Assuming you keep away from cheddar made with rennet, search for veggie lover Parmesan cheddar, which is made without it.

Nutrition Facts
(per serving)
402 Calories
22g Fat
37g Carbs
17g Protein

<u>Broccoli-Cheddar Soup</u>

Active Time:20 mins
Total Time:20 mins
Servings:4

Ingredients

- 1 tablespoon extra-virgin olive oil

- 1 cup chopped yellow onion

- 1 teaspoon minced garlic

- 3 cups lower-sodium vegetable broth

- ¼ teaspoon salt

- 3 cups broccoli florets, cut into 3/4-inch pieces

- ¾ cup matchstick carrots

- 2 cups whole milk

- 3 tablespoons cornstarch

- 2 cups finely shredded sharp Cheddar cheese

Directions

1. Heat oil in a huge Dutch broiler over medium intensity. Add onion; cook for about 4 minutes, stirring occasionally, until translucent. Add garlic; cook, blending continually, until fragrant, around 1 moment.

2. Add stock and salt; heat to the point of boiling over medium-high intensity. Add broccoli and carrots. Diminish intensity to keep a stew; cook, mixing periodically, until the vegetables are delicate, around 10 minutes.

3. In the meantime, whisk milk and cornstarch together in a fluid estimating cup; sprinkle into the soup, mixing continually. Cook, blending continually, until thickened, around 2 minutes. Eliminate from heat; step by step add Cheddar, blending until softened after every option

Nutrition Facts

(per serving)

398 Calories

26g Fat

23g Carbs

20g Protein

Red Curry-Coconut Soup

Active Time:40 mins
Total Time:50 mins
Servings:6

Ingredients

- 1 medium red onion

- 1 tablespoon unrefined coconut oil

- 1 small red bell pepper, finely chopped

- 1 tablespoon seeded and finely chopped jalapeño pepper, plus 2 tablespoons thinly sliced, divided

- 1 large sweet potato, scrubbed and chopped (about 4 cups)

- 1 tablespoon finely chopped garlic

- 1 tablespoon grated fresh ginger

- 3 tablespoons plus 1 teaspoon red curry paste

- 3/4 teaspoon salt

- 1/4 teaspoon ground pepper

- 4 cups lower-sodium chicken broth

- 1 (14-ounce) can coconut milk, well stirred

- 1 pound shredded cooked chicken breast (about 3 cups)

- 2 cups fresh green beans, trimmed and sliced into 1-inch pieces

- 1/2 cup finely chopped fresh cilantro

- 1/2 cup finely chopped fresh basil

- 1 tablespoon lime juice

Directions

1. Meagerly cut around one-fourth of onion to quantify 1/4 cup. Chop the remaining onion finely.

2. Dissolve coconut oil in a medium Dutch broiler over medium intensity. Add the slashed onion, ringer pepper and 1 tablespoon cleaved jalapeño; cook for about 2 minutes, stirring occasionally, until slightly softened. Add yam, garlic and ginger; cook, blending continually, until fragrant, around 1 moment. Add curry glue, salt and pepper; cook, blending continually, until the curry glue is fragrant and turns a couple of shades hazier, around 2 minutes.

3. Mix in stock and coconut milk; simmer for a few minutes over medium heat. Cover, and cook until the yam is practically delicate, around 10 minutes.

4. Mix in chicken and green beans. Cook, revealed, blending sporadically, until the beans are radiant green and delicate, around 10 minutes. Eliminate from heat; mix in cilantro, basil and lime juice.

5.   Split the soup between 6 dishes. Top with the saved cut onion and the excess 2 tablespoons of cut jalapeno.

Nutrition Facts
(per serving)
402 Calories
20g Fat
29g Carbs
29g Protein

Sausage, Tomato And White Bean Stew

Prep Time:15 mins
Additional Time:30 mins
Total Time:45 mins
Servings:4
Yield:4 servings

Ingredients

- 8 ounces sweet Italian turkey sausage, removed from casings

- ½ cup chopped onion

- 1 tablespoon olive oil

- 1 (28 ounce) can no-salt-added diced tomatoes

- 1 (15 ounce) can no-salt-added cannellini beans, drained and rinsed

- Freshly ground black pepper

- 3 cups baby spinach (3 ounces)

Directions

1. Cook the sausage and onion for about 6 minutes in hot oil in a large saucepan over medium heat until browned.

2. To the pot, add the beans, 1 cup of water, and the tomatoes. Season with pepper. Stew for 15 minutes. Add the spinach and cook until recently withered, around 1 moment.

Nutrition Facts
(per serving)
241 Calories
9g Fat
25g Carbs
16g Protein

Shrimp And Fish Stew

Active Time:30 mins
Total Time:30 mins
Servings:4
Yield:4 servings

Ingredients

- 8 ounces skinless cod or sea bass fillets

- 6 ounces raw shrimp (31-40 per pound), peeled and deveined

- ⅓ cup chopped onion

- 2 stalks celery, sliced

- ½ teaspoon minced garlic

- 2 teaspoons extra-virgin olive oil

- 1 cup reduced-sodium chicken broth

- ¼ cup dry white wine or reduced-sodium chicken broth

- 1 (14.5 ounce) can no-salt-added diced tomatoes, drained

- 1 (8 ounce) can no-salt-added tomato sauce

- 1 teaspoon dried oregano, crushed

- ¼ teaspoon salt

- ⅛ teaspoon ground black pepper

- 1 tablespoon snipped fresh parsley

Directions

1. Cut fish into 1 1/2-inch pieces. Split shrimp in half along their length. Refrigerate until prepared to utilize.

2. Heat oil in a huge pot over medium intensity. Add onion, celery, and garlic and cook, blending sometimes, until delicate, around 5 minutes. Cautiously mix in 1 cup stock and wine. Heat to the point of boiling. Diminish intensity to a stew and cook for 5 minutes. Mix in depleted tomatoes, pureed tomatoes, oregano, salt and pepper. Get back to a bubble, then, at that point, lessen intensity to a stew, cover and cook for 5 minutes.

3. Delicately mix in fish and shrimp. Get back to a bubble, then, at that point, quickly diminish intensity to low. Cover and stew until the fish drops effectively with a fork and the shrimp are hazy, 3 to 5 minutes. Sprinkle with parsley prior to serving.

Nutrition Facts
(per serving)
165 Calories
4g Fat
12g Carbs
19g Protein

Pork And Green Chile Stew

Prep Time:25 mins
Additional Time:4 hrs
Total Time:4 hrs 25 mins
Servings:6
Yield:6 servings

Ingredients

- 2 pounds boneless pork sirloin roast or shoulder roast

- 1 tablespoon vegetable oil

- ½ cup chopped onion (1 medium)

- 4 cups peeled and cubed potatoes (4 medium)

- 3 cups water

- 1 (15 ounce) can hominy or whole-kernel corn, drained

- 2 (4 ounce) cans diced green chile peppers, undrained

- 2 tablespoons quick-cooking tapioca

- 1 teaspoon garlic salt

- ½ teaspoon ground cumin

- ½ teaspoon ancho chile powder

- ½ teaspoon ground pepper

- ¼ teaspoon dried oregano, crushed

- 1 tablespoon Chopped fresh cilantro

Directions

1. Cut back excess from meat. Cut the meat into 1/2-inch pieces. Cook half of the meat in a huge skillet in hot oil over medium-high intensity until sautéed. Utilizing an opened spoon, eliminate the meat from the skillet. Rehash with the excess meat and the onion. Channel off fat. Move the entirety of the meat and the onion to a 3 1/2-to 4 1/2-quart slow cooker.

2. Mix in potatoes, the water, hominy, green chile peppers, custard, garlic salt, cumin, ancho chile powder, ground pepper, and oregano. Cook with a lid on for 7 to 8 hours on Low or 4 to 5 hours on High. Whenever wanted, embellish each presenting with cilantro.

Nutrition Facts
(per serving)
180 Calories
4g Fat
23g Carbs
15g Protein

<u>Vegetable Stew</u>

Prep Time: 20 mins
Additional Time:30 mins
Total Time:50 mins
Servings:6
Yield:6 servings

Ingredients

- 3 tablespoons unsalted butter

- 1 ½ cups chopped yellow onion (from 1 medium onion)

- 2 medium carrots, cut diagonally into 1 1/2-inch pieces (1 1/2 cups)

- 3 large garlic cloves, smashed

- 1 cup chopped portobello mushroom cap (from 1 large mushroom cap, gills removed)

- 1 cup sliced celery (from 2 large stalks)

- 4 (15 ounce) cans no-salt-added fire-roasted diced tomatoes

- 2 cups unsalted vegetable stock

- 1 ½ cups thawed frozen corn

- 6 ounces baby Yukon Gold potatoes (about 8 potatoes), halved

- 2 cups thawed frozen meatless burger crumbles (such as MorningStar Farm Grillers Crumbles)

- 1 cup thawed frozen cut green beans

- ¾ cup thawed frozen sweet peas

- 1 teaspoon kosher salt

- ½ teaspoon ground pepper

Directions
- Liquefy spread in a huge, weighty pot over medium-high intensity. Add onion, carrots and garlic; cook, mixing at times, until the onion is delicate, around 4 minutes. Add mushrooms and celery; cook, mixing once in a while, until the mushrooms begin to mellow, around 4 minutes. Corn, potatoes, tomatoes, and stock are added; heat to the point of boiling over high intensity, blending incidentally. Diminish intensity to medium-low; Cover and simmer for about 15 minutes until the potatoes are almost tender. Mix in meatless disintegrates, green beans, peas, salt and pepper; cover and cook until the potatoes are delicate, around 5 minutes.

Nutrition Facts
(per serving)
250 Calories
7g Fat
38g Carbs
15g Protein

Chicken Stew with Turnips And Mushrooms

Cook Time: 45 mins
Total Time:45 mins
Servings:6
Yield: 6 servings, about 1 1/3 cups each

Ingredients

- 1 ½ pounds boneless, skinless chicken breasts, trimmed

- ½ teaspoon salt, divided

- ¼ teaspoon freshly ground pepper

- 2 tablespoons extra-virgin olive oil, divided

- 2 large turnips (about 1 pound), peeled (see Tip) and cut into 1-inch pieces

- 8 ounces sliced cremini mushrooms

- 1 medium onion, sliced

- 2 cloves garlic, minced

- ½ cup dry white wine

- 4 cups chopped kale

- 3 cups reduced-sodium chicken broth

- 1 teaspoon fresh chopped rosemary

- 3 tablespoons cornstarch

- 3 tablespoons water

Directions

1. Slice chicken into 1-inch pieces and sprinkle with 1/4 teaspoon each salt and pepper.

2. Heat 1 tablespoon of oil in a Dutch stove over medium-high intensity. Add the chicken and cook, mixing regularly, until delicately sautéed, 3 to 4 minutes. Move to a plate.

3. Add the leftover 1 tablespoon of oil to the pot. Add turnips, mushrooms, onion and garlic and cook, blending every so often, until the onion is limp, 3 to 5 minutes. Add wine and cook, mixing, for 1 moment. Mix in kale, stock and rosemary. Return the chicken and any gathered juices to the pot; heat to the point of boiling. Lessen intensity to keep a stew, cover and cook, mixing more than once, until the turnips are delicate, around 10 minutes.

4. In the meantime, blend cornstarch and water in a little bowl. Mix the combination into the stew and cook until thickened, around 3 minutes. Season the stew with the remaining 1/4 teaspoon of salt after taking it off the heat.

Tips:

- Make certain to strip turnips well to eliminate all the toughness prior to cooking. To strip, slice off one finish to make a level surface so you can keep it consistent on the cutting board. Follow the shape of the vegetable with your blade to eliminate the skin. Or on the other hand, on the off chance that you utilize a vegetable peeler, strip around the root multiple times to eliminate all the stringy skin.

Nutrition Facts
(per serving)
242 Calories
8g Fat
13g Carbs
27g Protein

CHAPTER 10: **HEALTHY DRINKS AND BEVERAGES**

<u>Hearty Breakfast Smoothie</u>

Active Time:5 mins
Total Time:5 mins
Servings:1

Ingredients

- 1 medium banana (fresh or frozen)

- ½ cup sliced strawberries, blueberries or chopped mangos

- ¼ cup plain 2% Greek yogurt

- 1 tablespoon almond butter

- ½ cup baby spinach

- ½ cup unsweetened almond milk

- 1-2 basil leaves, 2-3 mint leaves or 1/2 teaspoon peeled, chopped ginger (optional)

Directions

- Place banana, strawberries (or blueberries or mango), yogurt, almond spread, spinach, almond milk and basil (or mint or ginger, if utilizing) in a blender; process until smooth.

Tips

- In the event that the smoothie is too thick, dainty it out with an extra sprinkle of almond milk. In the event that the smoothie is excessively slender, you can thicken it with a modest bunch of ice.

- For a dairy smoothie, use coconut milk yogurt instead of Greek yogurt. For a without nut smoothie, substitute ground flax seeds, sunflower seeds or pumpkin seeds for almond margarine.

Nutrition Facts
(per serving)
300 Calories
11g Fat
40g Carbs
13g Protein

Strawberry-Blueberry-Banana Smoothie

Prep Time: 5 mins
Total Time:5 mins
Servings:1
Yield:2 cups

Ingredients

- ½ cup frozen strawberries

- ½ cup frozen blueberries

- 1 small ripe banana (frozen, if desired)

- ¾ cup chilled unsweetened cashew milk, plus more if needed

- 1 tablespoon cashew butter

- 1 tablespoon hulled hemp seeds

Directions

- Join strawberries, blueberries, banana, cashew milk, cashew spread and hemp seeds in a blender. Process until smooth, adding more cashew milk, if necessary, for wanted consistency. Serve right away.

Nutrition Facts
(per serving)
335 Calories
17g Fat
46g Carbs
7g Protein

Anti-Inflammatory Beet Smoothie

Active Time: 5 mins
Total Time:5 mins
Servings:2

Ingredients
- 1 cup frozen strawberries

- 1 cup frozen blueberries

- 1 cup orange juice

- 1 (8.8-ounce) package refrigerated cooked beets (such as Love Beets)

- 1 medium banana, peeled

- 1 medium carrot, peeled and sliced

- 1 (1/2 inch) piece fresh ginger, peeled and grated

Directions
- Consolidate strawberries, blueberries, squeezed orange, beets, banana, carrot and ginger in a blender; process until consolidated, around 30 seconds. Split between 2 glasses. Serve right away.

Nutrition Facts
(per serving)
248 Calories
1g Fat

58g Carbs
4g Protein

Peanut Butter And Chocolate Banana Smoothie

Cook Time:5 mins
Total Time:5 mins
Servings:2
Yield:2 servings

Ingredients

- 1 cup nonfat milk

- 1 frozen medium banana

- 2 tablespoons natural peanut butter

- 1 tablespoon unsweetened cocoa powder

- 1 tablespoon chia or hemp seeds (optional)

- 1 teaspoon vanilla extract

Directions

Blend together milk, banana, peanut butter, chocolate, hemp or chia seeds (if desired), and vanilla. Blend until smooth.

Nutrition Facts

(per serving)
211 Calories
9g Fat
24g Carbs
9g Protein

Tomato-Vegetable Juice

Active Time:15 mins
Total Time:15 mins
Servings:2
Yield: 2 servings, about 8 ounces each

Ingredients

- 1 cup chopped hearts of romaine

- ¼ cup chopped fresh chives

- 2 large tomatoes, cut into wedges

- ¼ fresh jalapeno, stemmed and seeded

- 1 large red bell pepper, cut into eighths

- 2 large stalks celery, trimmed

- 1 medium carrot, peeled

- Ice cubes (Optional)

Directions

1. Working in a specific order, process romaine, chives, tomatoes, jalapeño, ringer pepper, celery and carrot through a juicer as per the maker's headings.

2. If you want, add ice to two glasses and pour the juice into them. Serve right away.

Nutrition Facts
(per serving)
46 Calories
9g Carbs
1g Protein

Ginger-Beet Juice

Active Time:15 mins
Total Time:15 mins
Servings:2
Yield: 2 servings, about 8 ounces each

Ingredients

- 1 medium orange, peeled and quartered

- 3 kale leaves

- 1 medium apple, cut into wedges

- 1 medium carrot, peeled

- 1 large beet, peeled and cut into wedges

- 1 1-inch piece peeled fresh ginger

- Ice cubes (optional)

Directions

1. Working in a specific order, process orange, kale, apple, carrot, beet and ginger through a juicer.

2. If you want, add ice to two glasses and pour the juice into them. Serve right away.

Nutrition Facts
(per serving)
100 Calories
1g Fat
21g Carbs
2g Protein

<u>**Lavender Latte**</u>

Active Time:10 mins
Total Time:40 mins
Servings:2

Ingredients

- ¼ cup granulated sugar

- ¼ cup water

- 2 tablespoons dried culinary lavender, plus more for garnish

- 1 ½ cups unsweetened plain barista-blend oat milk

- ⅔ cup hot strong brewed espresso blend coffee

Directions

1. Mix sugar, water and lavender together in a little pan; bring to a simmer in a large pot. Stew, blending periodically, until the sugar has disintegrated and the combination is fragrant, 1 to 2 minutes. Eliminate from heat; Allow it to steep for 30 minutes. Pour the combination through a fine-network sifter, disposing of solids; put the syrup away. Flush the pan.

2. Heat oat milk in the pan over medium-low intensity until it comes to 155°F to 165°F, 2 to 3 minutes. Empty the hot milk into a tall metal glass or other high-sided heat proof holder; Blend with a milk frother for about 30 seconds until bubbly and frothy.

3. Pour 1/3 mug espresso into every one of 2 (14-ounce) cups. Mix 2 teaspoons of the syrup into each mug. (Keep the remaining syrup in the fridge for later use.) Top each with half of the foamed milk. Embellish with extra lavender, whenever wanted..

Nutrition Facts
(per serving)
115 Calories
1g Fat
23g Carbs
3g Protein

Kitchen Tips And Tricks

Need a little assistance in the kitchen? While we can't offer you one more arrangement of hands or additional counter space, what about the following best? Whether you're an unbelievable home cook or a beginner, we ensure you'll need to take on in excess of a couple of these cooking tips. We offer kitchen strategies for further developing how you prep, cook, and store food as well as ways of making your kitchen apparatuses and contraptions turn out more enthusiastically for you. Tie your cover, focus in, and how about we go!

Step By Step Instructions To Keep Food From Staying

- Utilize a metal spatula to slacken the vegetables or meat, and afterward push them aside of the skillet.

- Slant the dish so the unfilled region is over the intensity.

- Add 1 to 2 tablespoons of oil to the unfilled region and allow it to get hot prior to moving the food back.

Restoring Solidified Honey

- To take honey back to a tasty, drizzly state: Place the compartment in a bowl of heated water until the honey is smooth and runny (5 to 10 minutes). On the other hand, eliminate the cover and microwave the container in 30-second stretches, checking after each.

- To keep precious stones from framing once more: Store the honey in a cool, dry spot (not the fridge) and try not to prevent dampness. That is, once your spoon touches your tea, you can't double dip.

Cutting Rolly-Polly Vegetables Securely

- To guard your fingers from scratches, utilize this method on round, shaky vegetables like potatoes, squash, and beets.

- With a sharp blade and a cutting board, cut a slender cut along the length of the vegetable to make a level side.

- Turn the veggie cut-side down on the cutting board (guaranteeing it's steady and won't roll away) and cut as wanted, halting when the veggie becomes shaky and hard to hold.

- Turn the veggie so the wide, level side from which you made the keep going cut is facedown on the cutting board, and afterward keep on cutting as wanted.

Mastering Whipped Cream

- Begin with the appropriate components. For feathery, stable whipped cream, use containers marked "weighty cream," "whipping cream," or "weighty whipping cream." (Save the light cream for espresso.) For pleasantness, add 2 tablespoons granulated sugar for some cream prior to beating.

- Observe cautiously. In a chilled bowl with an electric blender on high, beat chilled cream and sugar until the mixers leave noticeable lines when drawn across the cream. Lessen blender speed to medium-low and keep on beating until delicate pinnacles structure. (At the point when you hold up the blenders, the cream ought to stand up, and afterward the flop is finished.)

- Don't worry if you whip too hard. Using a rubber spatula, fold in a splash of fresh, unwhipped cream to the curdled lumps. Rehash depending on the situation until the combination smooths out.

A Cleaner Method For Breaking An Egg

- At the point when you tap a new egg on the edge of a bowl, you don't simply break the shell. The dainty film encompassing the white and the yolk likewise cracks, permitting little shell shards to blend in with the fluid and add an unwanted smash to your completed dish (most horrendously awful omelet fixing of all time).

- To make a single, clean break, crack the egg on a flat surface like a counter. Like that, the film stays in salvageable shape, meaning no shell in your scramble. Here is the procedure.

- Hold the egg in one hand and tap it immovably on a hard surface.

- Actually look at the break: You ought to see a space and one side-to-side break, similar to an equator.

- Put your thumbs on one or the other side of the break and delicately pull the shell separated. Any shards will adhere to the film, not fall into the bowl.

Taking Your Broiler's Temperature

- Stoves lie. Yours might say 350 degrees F, yet your last bunch of brownies was soft despite the fact that you followed the baking time. What gives? Sooner or later, broilers might lose precision, approaching 25 degrees off the set temperature. To test yours, follow these means.

- When the oven indicates that it has reached that temperature, place an oven-safe thermometer on the middle rack and heat the oven to 300 degrees.

- On the off chance that it peruses 275 degrees F, you know to consistently set the temperature 25 degrees higher. At the point when you become weary of figuring it out, look for an extremely durable fix by calling a repairman suggested by the maker.

The Most Effective Method To Cleave Garlic

- Love cooking with garlic yet disdain battling with tacky, paper-slender strips? With these three stages — trim, squash, cleave — you can prepare a clove quickly

- Cut off the hard root of each clove with the chef's knife's tip. This makes it easier for the skin to peel off.)

- With the blade pointing away from you, place a clove underneath the flat side of the knife. Press the impact point of your palm or your clench hand down on the blade until you feel the clove give way. Sneak off and dispose of the skin

- Accumulate the stripped cloves, hold your blade by the handle, and spot your other, nondominant hand on top of the cutting edge. Rock the blade all over through the cloves (with the tip remaining on the cutting board). Slash until the garlic is the size you need.

Removing Salmon Bones

- The backbone and ribs of a salmon are removed by a fishmonger prior to the salmon filets entering the seafood case at the supermarket.

However, they sometimes miss the soft, thin pin bones that "float" in the flesh. Here is a speedy method for eliminating them at home

- Run your forefinger along the middle crease of the filet, contradicting some common norms. On the off chance that there are any pin bones, you'll feel them jutting at about ½-inch span

- With clean tweezers, handle the tip of the bone and pull, pulling at a slight point rather than up and out. (Pin bones become skewed toward the fish's head.) Rehash as needs be.

Storing Tomato Paste Leftovers

- The majority of recipes that call for tomato paste, such as pesto, pasta sauce, and chili, only use a couple of tablespoons. In the event that your glue arrives in a cylinder, extras aren't an issue; in any case, on the off chance that it's in and would be able, don't throw the rest off to allow it to dry out in the cooler. Do this all things being equal.

- Spoon tablespoon-sized parts of tomato glue in an ice-block plate and spot it in the cooler.

- When strong, move the blocks to a plastic cooler sack.

- Utilize your frozen blocks of tomato glue straightforwardly in recipes; don't bother defrosting.

Keeping Prepared Merchandise New

- Most occasion treats, bars, and chomps keep going for as long as seven days in a firmly fixed compartment, yet imagine a scenario in which you're wanting to give them as a gift in an essential box.

Attempt this to keep up with newness until you drop them off to the fortunate beneficiary.

- The secret: Enclose the whole present by cling wrap or on the other hand, in the event that size permits, slip it into a resealable plastic pack. Your sweet treats will remain moist and chewy for days when they are shielded from the dry air.

Step By Step Instructions To Clean A Carefully Prepared Cast Iron Container

- With regards to cleaning a carefully prepared cast iron skillet, it's vital to not utilize cleanser or scouring powder, which will obliterate the non-stick covering. Do this all things considered

- the skillet with legitimate salt and scour it with a paper towel

- Wash the skillet clean under boiling water

- After thoroughly drying the pan with paper towels, apply a thin layer of vegetable oil

- In the event that you keep your cookware stacked, place a paper towel in the container to safeguard its surface.

CONCLUSION

As you arrive at the finish of this cookbook, we bid you a tasty goodbye, improved with the tempting smells and magnificent preferences you've found on each page. The culinary excursion imparted to Evelyn G. Powell has been in excess of an assortment of recipes; it's been a section through an existence where enthusiasm, imagination, and a guarantee to wellbeing entwine.

In each dish, Evelyn poured fixings as well as long periods of devotion, refining her specialty and building a sanctuary where the delight of cooking meets the quest for a better way of life. The pages turned were recipes as well as sections in a culinary story - a story of sizzles, blends, and the enchanted that happens when love is the primary fixing.

As you convey these recipes into your kitchen, may they flash satisfaction, rouse trial and error, and carry a bit of Evelyn's charm to your feasting table. Whether you're on a weight reduction venture or basically looking for flavorful, healthy feasts, this cookbook is your aide, and Evelyn is your culinary sidekick.

So here's to the craft of cooking, the delight of disclosure, and the flavors that make life a heavenly experience. May your kitchen continue to be a place where you can come up with new ideas, laugh, and, most importantly, make delicious food smell good.

Cheerful cooking, blissful living, and until we meet again on your next culinary Adventure!